COPING WITH PSORIASIS

DR RONALD MARKS is Professor of Dermatology at the University of Wales College of Medicine, Cardiff. He has lectured in many countries around the world, and has a special research interest in psoriasis. He has edited and contributed to several medical textbooks including *Investigative Techniques in Dermatology, Dermatology Postgraduate Tutorials* and *Measurements of the Physical Properties of the Skin.*

Dr Marks is active in his local branch of the Psoriasis Association and believes strongly in the importance of good communications between doctors, nurses and patients. His hobbies are art appreciation and playing squash.

Overcoming Common Problems Series

For a full list of titles please contact
Sheldon Press, Marylebone Road, London NW1 4DU

Overcoming Common Problems Series

Overcoming Common Problems Series

Overcoming Common Problems

COPING WITH PSORIASIS

Dr Ronald Marks

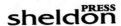

First published in 1981 by Martin Dunitz Limited

This new, fully-revised edition published in Great Britain in 1994
by Sheldon Press, SPCK, Marylebone Road, London NW1 4DU

Third impression 2000

British Library Cataloguing-in-Publication Data
A catalogue record for this book is available from the British Library
ISBN 0–85969–690–1

Photoset by Deltatype Ltd, Ellesmere Port, Cheshire
Printed in Great Britain by Biddles Ltd, www.biddles.co.uk

Contents

To Hilary for still putting up with me

Introduction

There are millions of men and women all over the world today who suffer from psoriasis. The latest surveys suggest that as many as two in every hundred of the total population have it at any one time. Yet psoriasis is a skin disease about which the public in general knows next to nothing. Inevitably, someone who has just been told for the first time that he or she has psoriasis is likely to have many questions to ask about it. What is it? Why did I develop it? Is it infectious? Will it spread? Will it go away? What kind of treatment is there for it? What can I do to help it?

Unfortunately, the busy family doctor tends to have far too little time to be able to satisfy his patients' desire for information and reassurance. Also, in many countries skin specialists (known as dermatologists) are still such a rarity that patients may have to face a long wait before they can see the person best qualified to answer all their questions. I hope this book will supply the information psoriasis sufferers need about the nature of their disease, and what it may mean to them in terms of their work, their leisure activities and their general health. It is certainly not intended to be a substitute for treatment by a doctor, but simply to explain, interest and reassure, as well as generally assist the process of recovery.

Psoriasis can be a very persistent complaint. It does not kill, but it is responsible for a great deal of unhappiness. Simply coping with the symptoms themselves can be a time-consuming and frustrating business, and many people with psoriasis will experience feelings of depression at some point. I hope that this book, without under-estimating the problems, will be able to put forward some constructive suggestions on how you can cope with them.

Among the everyday difficulties that someone with psoriasis must come to terms with is the way other people react to his condition. At the worst, they may recoil from it in fear and disgust – which is an understandable but very unhelpful primitive response to the sight of something abnormal. Gaining an understanding of the disease can do much to soften this harsh reaction, and so this book is intended for the family and friends of people with psoriasis no less than for the patients themselves.

Finally, I hope my book will be read by teachers, social workers and others whose work brings them into contact with people who suffer from psoriasis. These people will be in a much better position to offer help if they are aware of the career difficulties and social problems that psoriasis sufferers may come across as a result of their complaint. If it is also read by family doctors and officials concerned with allocating funds at a local or national level, so much the better.

Psoriasis is by no means a new disease. There are references to a skin disorder that sounds suspiciously like it in the Bible, although it seems likely that (as with many other skin diseases) people confused it with leprosy for a long time. In spite of its antiquity, it is a disease that has only fairly recently begun to be understood. Even now we still do not know the cause of psoriasis or why it persists, but painstaking research over the past thirty or forty years has solved many of the old mysteries about it. The seventh veil that obscures our final understanding is still intact, but with continued effort we may hope to see it lifted in the not too distant future.

In the dozen years or so that have sped by since I first wrote this book, many advances have occurred. These have made it necessary to update many sections. Although there have been several changes, the basic content is much the same, as sadly the underlying need still exists.

1
Ordinary Psoriasis

There are several different types of psoriasis, but far and away the most widespread is ordinary (or plaque-type) psoriasis. This accounts for about 95 per cent of all cases, and is the kind I shall mainly be concerned with. The other, very much rarer types are discussed separately in the next chapter.

How many people suffer from psoriasis?

Psoriasis is a very common problem. It is thought that as many as two per cent of the population suffer from it, although getting reliable statistics is not as easy as you might think.

Conducting a survey is a complicated business and, if the results are to be any good at all, many safeguards have to be built into it. First of all care has to be taken to make sure that the sample of people you examine is both random and typical. This is easier said than done where psoriasis is concerned. Even if we could just stop people in the street and ask them to slip their clothes off while we checked for psoriasis (and you can imagine what the response would be if we did!) we would also have to provide trained dermatologists to examine them. Otherwise mistakes would be made in identifying which of them had psoriasis and which hadn't. If the diagnosis wasn't right the survey would end up with quite false conclusions.

In spite of all the problems, some excellent surveys have been carried out in Sweden, Britain, the United States and in the Faeroe Isles off the coast of Denmark. These all support the theory that between one and two per cent of the population have psoriasis at the time that any one survey is made. Similar tests carried out in Japan and West Africa suggest that psoriasis may be rather less common in these countries, but that even so it still affects a significant section of the population.

Obviously, the number of people who suffer from psoriasis at some point in their lives will be larger than the number who have it at any one time. Unfortunately we don't have any reliable figures that could tell us just what proportion of the population suffer from psoriasis at some stage during their passage from cradle to grave.

We do know roughly how many of the people who are referred to outpatient departments for skin disease have psoriasis. It seems to be about six per cent of all new patients seen at skin clinics. When you start investigating how many of the people going back for repeat visits have psoriasis the proportion is much higher, since many other skin diseases only need one or two visits to the clinic. These statistics about outpatients are not completely reliable, as several factors can distort the picture they give. For example the reputation of the hospital, the structure of the population in the area and the willingness of the local doctors to refer their patients to the hospital can all affect the figures.

Statistics like these cannot of course give us any indication of how a particular case of psoriasis will behave, and they only tell us about how many people suffer from it, not about how severe a problem it is or how long it lasts. But what does emerge clearly from all the research is that psoriasis is a disease of major importance to the community. When you know that there are, for example, as many as a million sufferers in Britain, and four million in the United States, you begin to realize that it is a problem that deserves to be taken seriously.

Who is most likely to get psoriasis?

It would be interesting if we were able to link psoriasis with factors such as social background or your job, but in general we can't. The only exception appears to be that butchers and people whose work involves contact with animal skins may be particularly likely to develop psoriasis. This rather curious fact would seem to be fertile ground for research, but I know of no work going on at the moment to confirm this or to investigate it further.

It seems also that slightly more men than women get psoriasis. Husbands or wives of people with psoriasis are statistically more likely than other people to have the condition, but the reason for this could be that people tend to group together and meet with others who have the same problem.

Psoriasis does seem to run in families to some extent, and if your parents or other relatives suffer from it you stand a markedly increased risk of developing the disease. The role of heredity in psoriasis is discussed in greater detail on page 26.

The most common age for someone to develop psoriasis is during their teens or twenties, but it can appear at any age. There is another main 'danger period' later in life, when you are in your fifties and sixties. It is quite common for people who have been free of all signs of psoriasis suddenly to have their first attack of it at this age. Early onset psoriasis is known as Type 1 psoriasis and that starting later in life is known as Type 2.

What does common psoriasis look like?

Common or plaque-type psoriasis gets its name from the appearance of the patches of affected skin. Each patch looks like a plaque or small disc stuck onto the surface of the body. The patches of abnormal skin are often a dull red wine colour but may be a brighter shade of red and they stand out sharply from the apparently normal skin surrounding them. They are often rounded or oval in shape, or they may have an irregular outline which sometimes looks as though several rounded patches have joined up together.

The surface of each patch of psoriasis is rough to touch and has a scaly appearance. How scaly it is depends on several factors, including how long the patch has been there, what treatment it has received and where it is. It is easy to make a patch of psoriasis look less scaly for a few minutes – just wet it! Moisturizing creams make psoriasis look less scaly for about half an hour but take about the same amount of time to work. The scale has sometimes been described as looking silvery and rather like candle grease. It tends to be worse on patches of psoriasis over the legs, knees, elbows and scalp, and generally improves with treatment quickly.

How is it different from other skin conditions?

It is not much good treating someone for psoriasis if what they have really got is eczema. Different skin diseases respond to different drugs. Not all that is red and scaly is psoriasis. And although most people with common psoriasis have a rash that is easily identifiable, in other cases it can be quite difficult for a doctor to get the diagnosis right first time, even if he is a dermatologist with special experience of skin diseases.

The condition that is most often confused with psoriasis is eczema. From the patient's point of view the main difference between the two rashes is that eczema is usually itchy and psoriasis usually isn't. But some people with psoriasis are unlucky enough to have itchy patches too, so a doctor cannot go by this alone. Psoriasis patches tend to have quite sharply defined borders, but areas of eczema generally do not.

Another rash that can resemble psoriasis is called ringworm. This is the result of a particular kind of fungus infection. Patches of ringworm tend to occur singly rather than in several typical sites as psoriasis patches do, and, not surprisingly in view of the name, are often ring shaped.

There are several other skin diseases that can look like psoriasis, but most of them are too uncommon to be worth describing here. One is the amazingly named pityriasis rubra pilaris, usually shortened to PRP. This can certainly look quite like common psoriasis, but it tends to be a slightly different colour and to affect the hair follicles particularly, which is not true of psoriasis.

Special tests for psoriasis

In most cases your doctor will be able to tell definitely whether or not you have psoriasis on the basis of the distinctive appearance and history of your skin problem. But occasionally, if he is not quite sure, he may want to carry out special tests to find out exactly what the trouble is. The tests in common use are simple, informative, quick and not at all unpleasant.

One test that the doctor may use to find out whether you have got a ringworm infection is to scrape some of the scales off a patch and examine them through a microscope where the fungus responsible for ringworm will show up.

If the doctor thinks that the rash may be caused by eczema, and might be the result of an allergy, he may arrange for you to have a patch test. When this happens, sticky plasters containing substances to which you might be allergic are applied to your skin (usually on your back). If you are allergic to any of the substances, a rash will develop after about 48 hours at the place where the patch was applied.

If these tests do not supply a clear answer, the doctor may want to remove a small piece of the abnormal skin, so that it can be examined under a microscope. This is known as a biopsy. It is a very simple procedure, usually carried out in a hospital outpatient department or health centre, and is quite safe. First of all the area from which the skin is to be removed is numbed by injecting a local anaesthetic into it. Once this has taken effect, a small piece of skin is cut away, and a few stiches inserted to close the wound if necessary. The whole process usually takes no more than five or ten minutes.

A biopsy is certainly nothing to be frightened about, although it may leave a small scar behind. I have had several biopsies myself, and I can honestly say that I would rather have ten of them than have one tooth filled.

Occasionally a dermatologist may suggest other tests if he feels that your general health is either causing the skin complaint or suffering as a result of it. Blood tests and urine tests are both ways of checking up on this. Most people have experienced these tests at some stage and will be aware that they are nothing to worry about.

The tests I have been describing are really the exception rather than the rule, as in most cases common psoriasis is not difficult to identify. Your doctor is more likely to need this sort of test to help diagnose the rarer types of rash described in the next chapter.

How psoriasis develops

Generally speaking each spot of psoriasis starts life as a small reddened area that gradually gets bigger by spreading outwards. The spot may be any size from pinhead upwards. Sometimes people start with two or three patches and then a few more appear elsewhere, or the original spots just grow larger. After a while the spots stop expanding and stay the same size for some time. This is called the stable phase, and generally occurs after a few weeks, although it does vary from one person to another. How large the spot grows before reaching the stable phase is also something that varies greatly, but an average size might be anything from two to three inches (5 to 8 cm) across. Uncommonly the patches appear suddenly over a few days – almost like measles or chicken pox.

The patch of stable psoriasis may eventually start to grow paler and less scaly until it disappears altogether. However, it is just as possible for it to begin to enlarge again for no obvious reason. Even if a patch in one particular place does fade away completely, it may be reactivated later on and reappear in the same way as it did before.

Which parts of the body are most often affected?

The elbows, knees, scalp and the lower back are the areas most frequently affected. The patches may appear in other places as well but the face, hands and feet are not often affected by common psoriasis. Almost anywhere can be affected, but luckily most patients only develop a few patches.

In a few cases it seems to occur symmetrically – that is, people find that a patch on one side of the body is matched by one in the same place on the other side. But, although this happens more often than could be explained simply by chance, it is not the general rule and you are more likely to find that the patches are spread out in a quite random way.

About 50 per cent of people with psoriasis find that the condition spreads to their scalps, and this can be one of the most upsetting aspects of it. Most people will only get a few scaly areas on their heads, and these can often be coped with fairly easily along the lines suggested in chapter ten. In some cases, however, the scalp is more severely affected and thick crusty patches appear which are difficult to hide. Luckily these do not cause baldness, although there may be some slight temporary increased rate of hair loss. People severely affected by psoriasis of the scalp sometimes describe it by saying 'my head feels as if it is cased in concrete'. Fortunately treatment can do a lot to ease the discomfort. The snowstorms of white, dandruff-like flakes that the condition tends to cause, and that are often embarrassing, also respond well to treatment.

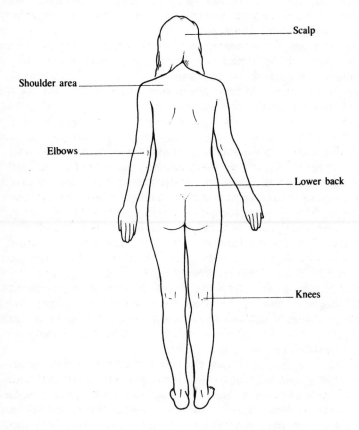

Figure 1. *Places on the body most often affected by common psoriasis*

Many people notice that when their psoriasis is on the rampage (as it will be from time to time) patches break out at any part of the body where they get a scratch or a minor injury. At the moment, as with so much about psoriasis, we still don't have an explanation as to why this happens.

How much discomfort does it cause?

Psoriasis is annoying mainly because of its unsightly appearance and its tendency to return again and again. It is not usually painful, except when uncommonly the palms and soles of the feet are affected and develop cracks. A vague feeling of discomfort or soreness may accompany psoriasis, but this again is more often a feature of the rarer kinds such as flexural psoriasis (see page 11) than of the common variety.

A few people find that their psoriasis is itchy, but they are very much the minority. Ordinary psoriasis is not normally an itchy complaint. Indeed the fact that it doesn't usually itch is one of the features that helps doctors to distinguish it from other skin problems such as eczema.

Will it go away?

One of the most annoying things for someone with psoriasis is that it is so unpredictable. It is very difficult for a doctor to forecast how psoriasis will behave for any particular person. Most doctors have some patients with small, unobtrusive patches of psoriasis on their knees or elbows which remain unchanged for ten, twenty, thirty years or even longer. These people may carry their patches of psoriasis to the grave without ever experiencing any problems from them. In other cases people who start off with exactly the same type of patches find, for no discernible reason, that they suddenly develop more and more of them, until the psoriasis covers large parts of their body. By the same token, even quite widespread psoriasis may suddenly fade away and disappear without any treatment at all. The only thing really predictable about psoriasis is its unpredictability!

The whole process varies so widely from one individual to another that it is very difficult for me to lay down any general rules about how it is likely to behave. But it is true to say that most people with psoriasis find that their symptoms are mild and persistent. In other words, once the disease has appeared it stays with them, in a not too serious form, getting periodically better and then worse. The patches often tend to break out suddenly at irregular intervals. Occasionally there will be a phase when the psoriasis goes on the rampage and many spots appear. But there will probably also be many quiet periods when the skin looks normal. Luckily in most cases people tend to find that the episodes when their psoriasis is being troublesome are quite short, with very much longer periods in between when they are relatively free from it. A few patients with psoriasis say that they are worse in the winter time, in the spring time, or some other season. Some others state that stress or other upset brings out psoriatic patches.

There are various forms of psoriasis that cause more problems than this, but most are quite rare. Some of them are variations on ordinary psoriasis, such as flexural (which is when psoriasis occurs in the creases of the body), guttate (which means that it appears as lots of tiny spots) or generalized (which is when the psoriasis covers the whole of your body). These and other unusual forms of psoriasis are all discussed in the next chapter.

2

Less Common Types of Psoriasis

Around one person in twenty with psoriasis has one of the less common forms of the disease. Some of these forms bear a resemblance to common psoriasis, but some of them are so different that only a doctor with wide experience of treating skin diseases will be able to recognize them as psoriasis. Indeed there is a certain amount of dispute among doctors about whether or not some of the conditions described in this chapter actually are types of psoriasis or some other sort of skin disorder. For the sake of completeness I have included all the problems that are frequently grouped together as variations of this one disease.

Flexural psoriasis (in the creases of the body)

This is the least unusual sort of the uncommon types of psoriasis. The only difference between it and ordinary psoriasis is that the patches, instead of being on the knees, elbows, back and so forth, are found in the folds and creases of the body. It is very rare for someone to have just flexural psoriasis, but people with ordinary psoriasis sometimes get one or two patches in the folded parts of their skin as well. It mainly affects people who are in their mid-forties or older, and particularly if they are overweight as this means they have more folds in their body.

Patches of flexural psoriasis tend to be moist rather than scaly. This is probably just the result of where they are. They can be more uncomfortable than patches of common psoriasis, and people with flexural psoriasis may feel quite sore in the affected areas. Occasionally they may also develop scaly patches round their eyes, ears and nose.

Guttate psoriasis (small, scattered spots)

This slightly odd name comes from the Latin word *gutta*, meaning a drop, and people suffering from it look as though their skin has been sprayed with drops from a paintbrush. Each spot is a mini version of the plaques of ordinary psoriasis. The difference is that the spots are much smaller and there are many more of them. Cases of guttate

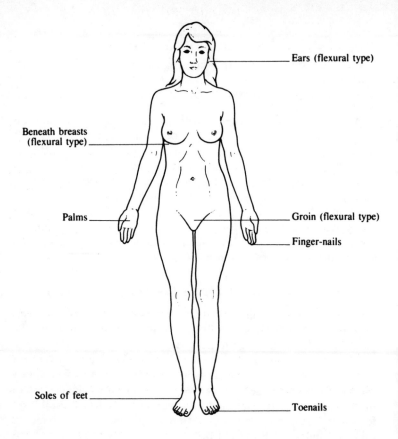

Figure 2. *Areas of the body affected by the less common forms of psoriasis*

psoriasis don't crop up very often – I see perhaps fifteen people or so with it every year. They are mainly youngsters between ages of eight and sixteen, and this again marks it out from ordinary psoriasis which rarely affects children.

Guttate psoriasis usually comes on quite suddenly, about two to four weeks after a sore throat. One particular type of sore throat known as streptococcal tonsillitis seems especially likely to be followed by guttate psoriasis, but we don't know why this should be so. The spots usually clear up by themselves after a few weeks, but in some cases they may linger on and eventually develop into larger patches of psoriasis.

Generalized psoriasis (all over the body)

This sort of psoriasis (which is also sometimes known as erythro-dermic psoriasis) is luckily very uncommon. As its name suggests it is a condition in which the patches of psoriasis spread all over the whole body. This may happen suddenly out of the blue and for no apparent reason, or it may develop gradually in someone who has had ordinary psoriasis for some time.

Generalized psoriasis looks less scaly than the plaques of common psoriasis, and the most striking feature of the skin may be that it turns very red more or less all over. This inflammation leads to various problems, as it can make you lose a lot of water through the skin, and also make you lose heat very easily (see page 22). It can be a disagreeable illness and make you feel thoroughly unwell. Because the patches of affected skin are so widespread it is often impractical to try treating it with creams and lotions, so your doctor is more likely to use medicines to control it (see page 49).

Psoriasis of the nails

This usually appears in individuals with ordinary psoriasis, but I include it here because it can also occur on its own, without the rest of the skin being affected.

Psoriasis can have several different effects on the fingernails and toenails. One person's nails may react differently from another's; the same person's nails may react differently at different times and it is quite common for different nails to be affected at different times in the same person.

One typical change is for the fingernails to become pitted. There will be a series of quite large dents (about 1 or 2 mm across) spread quite regularly over the surface of the nail. This type of reaction is sometimes described as 'thimble pitting' because it makes the surface of the nail look like the outside of a thimble.

Another thing that happens quite commonly is for the nail to separate slightly from the underlying nail bed (this is known in medical terms as onycholysis, and can happen as a result of several other diseases as well as psoriasis).

Sometimes nails will change colour as a result of psoriasis. If the nail becomes separated from its bed in the way I have just mentioned, a salmon pink patch may be visible on it. Occasionally the nail may become infected and then it will go a brown or greenish-black colour.

Toenails as well as fingernails can be affected by psoriasis, but

13

they tend to react by thickening, rather than in the ways I have been describing. In this case the nails may look rather as though they are suffering from a fungus infection, even though they are not.

Creams and ointments do not help much for psoriasis of the nails but in recent years some newer, more successful treatments have been developed. Sometimes you can be given injections around the nail. The problem tends to get better as the patches of psoriasis do.

Pustular psoriasis

This is something of a general description for several similar conditions. Most of these disorders are uncommon and this is just as well, as in general they are more unpleasant and cause more difficulties than ordinary psoriasis. Pustular psoriasis tends not to look quite like ordinary psoriasis although in some sufferers the ordinary and pustular forms may coexist, or one may follow the other.

The main distinguishing feature of pustular psoriasis is the appearance of pus spots (or pustules). These do not, as one might suppose, mean that any infection is present. They simply show that the skin has been invaded by the same white blood cells that would be seen if there were an infection. (In fact, this is something that happens to a limited extent with all types of psoriasis as I shall explain in the next chapter.)

The commonest type of pustular psoriasis occurs on the palms of the hands and the soles of the feet. Instead of the reddish patches you get from common psoriasis, in this condition you get white or yellow pus spots, which turn a darker yellow after a few days and eventually go brown and drop off. There is some dispute as to whether this is really a type of psoriasis or not.

If common psoriasis is treated with drugs known as corticosteroids (see page 44), pustules will sometimes appear on top of the patch of ordinary psoriasis. The pustules behave in just the same way as those described in the previous paragraph and, with treatment, they should eventually disappear. This not only applies to treatment with corticosteroids taken by mouth but also to treatment with some powerful corticosteroids in creams and ointments. There have been no proper surveys to assess the frequency of this complication, but it has undoubtedly become more common with increasing use of these preparations. It may well be that it is much more frequent in some countries than others because of the different usage of these treatments.

Another, and even rarer, complaint is generalized pustular

psoriasis (also known as von Zumbusch's disease, after the physican who first described it). Here the pustules occur all over the body, producing an unpleasant illness which is often accompanied by fever and joint pains. This is a more serious disease and usually needs hospital treatment.

I must emphasize again that the forms of psoriasis described in this chapter are exceptional. They are much rarer than ordinary psoriasis and do, on the whole, cause more trouble. It is these diseases, rather than the usual mild form, that are more likely to have the sort of repercussions on your general health described in chapter four. But clearly the most direct effects of psoriasis, of whatever kind, are the changes it makes to the skin. This is the first thing to consider when building up an understanding of the condition and I shall discuss it in the next chapter before going on to the more general problems associated with severe psoriasis.

Nappy or diaper psoriasis

This condition, which may not really by psoriasis at all, occurs in the nappy or diaper area of young infants. The areas affected can look as though they were affected by patches of ordinary psoriasis. The skin has the same dull red colour, and there is the same type of coarse scale on the surface. There is usually a sharp but irregular margin to the rash, and patches may spread to other parts of the child's body, particularly to the scalp or to the moist folds of skin such as those in the groin or under the arms. We do not know what causes it, and indeed, as I have mentioned, it may not be a type of psoriasis at all. It could be a kind of eczema or a reaction to an infection known as thrush – although few dermatologists hold this view today.

Parents tend to be understandably distressed by the appearance of this problem. But they may be reassured to know that the patches usually clear up quickly with treatment. If you take care to avoid irritating the area unnecessarily and apply bland creams prescribed by your doctor this will probably be enough to cope with the problem.

The other common fear parents have is that, after having nappy psoriasis, the child will go on to develop true psoriasis later in life. Further research is needed into whether or how these two may be connected, but so far it does not seem that a child who has had nappy psoriasis is at any added risk of going on to get another form of the disease.

3

What Happens to Your Skin if You Get Psoriasis

Most people give very little thought to how their skin works. In fact it is one of our most interesting organs and it carries out several very important functions. Among other things, it acts as a protective barrier and helps to regulate the temperature of our bodies. Healthy skin performs these roles with great efficiency. But when the skin is affected by psoriasis, several changes take place and affect its behaviour.

How your skin works

Normal skin can be thought of as having two parts – a tough, elastic inner layer called the dermis, and a thinner outer layer called the epidermis. This is not something you can tell just by looking at your skin, but the two layers are quite distinguishable when looked at under a microscope. (Incidentally, the old idea that skin is made up of seven layers is a complete myth.)

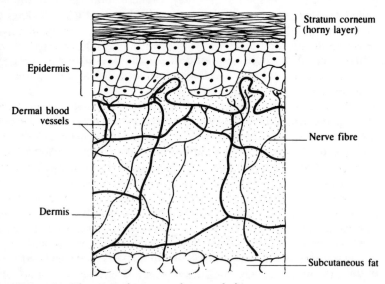

Figure 3. *The main features of normal skin*

16

The dermis is composed of the same sort of tissue as our ligaments and tendons. Within this layer are the nerves and tiny blood vessels (or capillaries) that supply our skin with food and oxygen, and also the tough fibres (known as the collagen) that give healthy skin its suppleness and elasticity.

The epidermis is made up of lots of oval or cube-shaped cells that are produced at its base (known as the basal cell layer). These move gradually up through the epidermis and become cells of the horny protective layer on the surface, and are ultimately shed. It normally takes around a month for a new cell in the basal layer to migrate up to the outer horny part of the epidermis and drop off. There are also tiny openings in the epidermis (our pores), and it is through some of these that we sweat as one way of lowering our body temperature when we are too hot. Other pores open into the hair follicles, which contain the growing parts of the hairs and the first part of the hairs themselves.

What changes occur when you get psoriasis

Psoriasis affects this general picture in several ways, the most typical of which is that it makes the epidermis grow thicker. You can sometimes notice this thickening from the way that a patch of psoriasis stands out as a slightly raised patch or plaque from the rest of your skin.

Two factors seem to contribute to this thickening. First, and most important, there is a huge increase in the basic number of cells within the epidermis. Secondly, fluid and blood cells accumulate in this layer. The whole epidermis becomes more folded than usual (see diagram), which is something you can see through a microscope but not with the naked eye.

There are also a number of changes that occur to the dermis (the lower layer of skin) when you get psoriasis. One thing that happens is that the blood vessels become more folded and much wider than normal, and the blood within them flows unusually rapidly. This increase in the blood supply to your skin explains why patches of psoriasis are red and why they bleed particularly easily.

Another change is that there are also an unusually high number of white blood cells in the dermis. This happens whenever your skin is inflamed for any reason, but what is unusual in the case of psoriasis is that some of these white blood cells move outwards and find their way into the outer layers of the skin. In pustular psoriasis (see page 14) the epidermis may not thicken as much as it does in common psoriasis, but there is more inflammation. The collections of these

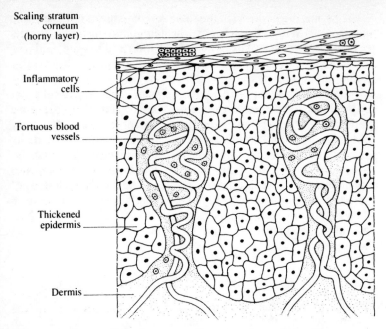

Scaling stratum corneum (horny layer)

Inflammatory cells

Tortuous blood vessels

Thickened epidermis

Dermis

Figure 4. *Some of the important features of psoriatic skin*

white cells form small 'abscesses', which account for the tiny pus spots that patients with this kind of psoriasis tend to have. In other kinds of psoriasis you cannot actually see that the white cells have moved to the outside of the skin unless you examine samples of skin under a microscope.

Why the skin goes scaly

The skin cells in patches of psoriasis grow very much more quickly than they do in normal skin. They also move upwards faster through the epidermis. In an area of skin affected by psoriasis a new cell may take only four days, instead of the normal twenty-eight, to move from the basal layer up to the outer surface. In other words the upward movement of the cells is about seven times faster than normal, and the cells on the surface are still very new. Young cells are more 'sticky' than old ones, which is why the scale is produced.

This rapid growth seems to be due to two things. First, as I have just described, there are a larger number of cells there to start with, and, second, there is an increase in the rate at which they divide. The rates can differ from one patch to another, or even within the same patch.

This high rate of growth is undoubtedly a very important element in psoriasis. Some researchers even claim that it is the basic cause of the disease, but it would seem more likely that it is a symptom than a cause. An abnormally high growth rate occurs in the cells of the epidermis whenever we injure our skin, and it seems to be a feature of other skin problems such as eczema as well as psoriasis. This, together with the fact that the increased rate of growth can be so variable, suggests that the extra cell growth is the result of the psoriasis, not the other way round.

In spite of the fact that I do not think this rapid cell growth is the direct cause of psoriasis, it would still be helpful to discover why the cells should grow so quickly. The knowledge could certainly provide an important link in the chain leading to the development of new kinds of treatment.

Changes in the way your skin behaves

The outer layer of our skin is usually an excellent protective barrier, keeping the body's fluids in and harmful substances and microbes out. But if you have psoriasis the barrier becomes much less effective.

One result of this is that water from the tissues in the skin seeps out and evaporates into the surrounding air much quicker than usual. In fact, depending on how severe your psoriasis is, the water can escape anything from three to ten times as fast as it does in normal skin. If only a small area of your skin is affected this does not matter much, but if you have severe and widespread psoriasis the water loss may be surprisingly high. As a result you may start to notice signs of dehydration, such as getting a dry skin and tongue, or feeling unusually thirsty.

As well as letting water out more easily, skin which is affected by psoriasis also allows substances to penetrate into it more easily than normal skin. This fact can be turned to your advantage. It means that any drugs you put on in the form of creams, lotions or ointments will work particularly well because they will be quickly and easily absorbed. Sometimes harmful bacteria live and multiply within the scales of psoriasis but in general patches of psoriasis don't get infected. Under certain special circumstances these bacteria could act as a source of infection that could be transferred to other people. For example, an anaesthetist with psoriasis might harbour bacteria that could contaminate surgical wounds during an operation. However, I must emphasize that this is extremely uncommon. For the most part people with psoriasis do not carry any infections at all.

One other effect of the changes in the horny layer of skin is that it loses much of its pliability and toughness. As a consequence cracks may develop on a patch of psoriasis, particularly in areas where the skin needs to be very flexible such as the palms of the hands or the soles of the feet. Cracks in these places can be painful and also a nuisance as they may make it difficult for you to walk comfortably or to use your hands for work.

Does psoriasis only affect the visible areas of skin?

To the naked eye, patches of psoriasis look quite clearly marked off from the skin that surrounds them. But under a microscope you can see that in fact the epidermis also thickens in the completely normal-looking skin that surrounds the patches.

The cells in these areas grow faster than usual, although not as fast as in the patch itself, and the outer layer of skin behaves in an abnormal way. It is less efficient at keeping water in than ordinary skin and the cells and blood vessels also show some signs of behaving in an unusual way. The closer to the patch of psoriasis you get, the more noticeable these abnormalities are in the apparently unaffected skin.

This is a subject into which intensive research has been going on for some years. Several questions are yet to be answered. I suppose the most important issue is whether someone who develops psoriasis in fact has abnormal skin from birth. If this turned out to be true, we might be able to predict early on whether a particular person was likely to get psoriasis later in life.

It would also be useful to know whether treatment affects these changes in the 'normal' skin, and whether they might continue, or come back, even after the actual patches of psoriasis had disappeared. This kind of study could give researchers a valuable guide towards understanding exactly what psoriasis does to the skin.

Because skin is such an important part of our bodies, any changes in the way it behaves can also have a few wider reaching influences on our health. Having looked at what happens to the skin itself I shall now go on to discuss some of the other problems that people with widespread psoriasis sometimes have.

4

How Severe Psoriasis Can Affect Your Health

Basically psoriasis is a condition that only affects patches of skin and does not cause ill health in any more general sense. Dermatologists often try to reassure their patients by telling them something like 'people with psoriasis are generally healthier than those with normal skin'. This well-meant offering is generally rather poorly received by the patient, but in one important sense it is true. The appearance of psoriasis does not usually have any serious significance so far as the rest of your health is concerned. The fact that someone develops the condition does not imply, as some skin disorders do, that he or she is likely to get any other associated disease such as diabetes, asthma or tuberculosis.

There are however a few, mainly minor, ways in which your health may suffer as a result of psoriasis and I shall discuss these, and ways in which you can cope with them, in this chapter. The most unpleasant effect is the form of arthritis discussed on page 22. This may crop up in, perhaps, five per cent of people with psoriasis. Like most of the other health problems I am going to describe it is really only likely to afflict you if you suffer from quite severe psoriasis. If your condition is mild and only affects a few parts of your body you should not have trouble with any of the difficulties discussed below.

Does psoriasis of the scalp affect your hair?

Even if you have quite bad psoriasis on your scalp, your hair itself is not usually affected. The disease does not make you go bald, or change the rate as which your hair grows. The scale over your hair can change slightly as a result of psoriasis, and sometimes more hair falls out than usual – but this loss is not permanent and it grows back again later. Some research work is going on to try to clarify our picture of exactly what effect psoriasis has on the hair, but the sort of changes it produces are not usually noticeable and do not cause major problems to most sufferers.

How psoriasis can affect body temperature

As I have explained, the flow of blood through the blood vessels is faster in a patch of psoriasis than in normal skin. This increased supply of blood makes the skin look and feel warmer than normal, but because the blood vessels are closer to the cooler air outside the body, the heat is lost more quickly. This means that although the skin will look and feel abnormally hot, the patient himself, in severe cases of psoriasis, may actually feel cold and shivery.

If the psoriasis is very widespread this kind of heat loss can occasionally produce a small but significant drop in body temperature – a state known as hypothermia. For this reason people with bad psoriasis should always be kept warm. This was something that was not always recognized in the past and tragedies sometimes occurred because people assumed that the psoriasis patient's red skin should be cooled down rather than heated up.

Psoriasis can also affect heat regulation in the opposite way. It sometimes happens that the scale you get on a patch of psoriasis can block up the openings in the skin through which we sweat (the pores). Sweating is one of the ways the body uses to cool down, and so this reduced ability to sweat can be a problem in a hot climate, or when you have 'flu or some other feverish illness. In these situations someone who has severe, widespread psoriasis may find that his body temperature soars to alarming heights. If so, it is of course important to cool him or her down by such methods as sponging the body with cold water or applying ice packs.

Arthritis

It is difficult to know just how prevalent arthritis (inflammation of the joints) is among people with psoriasis. Most surveys indicate that about one person in twenty with psoriasis has some form of arthritis and that about one person in twenty with arthritis has some form of psoriasis! However, these figures may be biased by the ways that the surveys have been conducted and the populations examined. It is certainly not most dermatologists' experience that one in twenty of their patients has severe arthritis. It may be that one in twenty has had some type of arthritis at some time. Luckily only a very small proportion of patients have a severe problem with their joints.

One sort of arthritis, called psoriatic arthropathy, only affects those with psoriasis. The disease most often attacks the joints at the ends of the fingers, which become swollen and painful. The jaw joints near the ears and some of the smaller joints of the back are sometimes also affected. In a small number of cases this disease can be very distressing. If it is allowed to progress unchecked it can eventually damage or even destroy the bone surfaces of the joints involved and, for example, make the fingers shorter. Fortunately this is extremely uncommon and can be greatly helped if the disease is properly treated in the early stages.

Another joint disease that psoriasis patients are more liable to get than most people is a kind of rheumatoid arthritis. It attacks the middle joints of the fingers (but not the end ones as in psoriatic arthropathy), and some larger joints such as the wrists and ankles. Very rarely it may also affect the hips. Laboratory tests can help distinguish this disease from ordinary rheumatoid arthritis, but from the patient's point of view the symptoms are very much the same. The joints become swollen and tender and do not work as well as they used to. The disease tends to flare up and then die down again in an unpredictable way and may, with luck, eventually burn itself out. There are no magic cures, but it can be helped with drugs and physiotherapy following the advice of your doctor.

Other rare problems sometimes associated with psoriasis

Circulation problems

If a great deal of your body's surface is covered with psoriasis this will make an extra demand on your blood circulation. In order to meet this demand and still maintain the blood supply to vital organs such as the brain and kidneys, the heart then has to work harder. Usually this does not cause any problems, and it can take on the extra load without difficulty. But if the patient has a problem with the blood vessels (such as hardening of the coronary blood vessels of the heart), his heart may be unable to perform this extra work adequately, and as a result he may feel out of breath. Anyone who gets out of breath after little or no exertion (whether or not this is the result of psoriasis) should of course see a doctor.

Swollen ankles

This can also be a sign that your heart is not strong enough to cope with the extra work produced by widespread psoriasis, so if your ankles do swell it makes sense to check up with your doctor about the problem.

People with severe generalized psoriasis, sometimes get swollen ankles even though they are otherwise perfectly healthy and have no heart problems at all. In this case the increased flow of blood to the skin and the slight leakiness of the blood vessels produced by psoriasis have changed the pressure in the blood vessels which in turn has caused the swelling. Once again, this is an uncommon problem and one you should raise with your own doctor.

Protein and mineral deficiency

These are rarely due to psoriasis, and only arise if someone has active disease over most of the body surface. It happens because the increased rate at which the skin cells grow and are shed may lead to a significant loss of protein and other essential chemicals from the body. Unless the patient makes good the loss he can go on to develop a type of anemia, or some other state of deficiency. In those rare instances where there is any risk of this, the doctor will generally advise the person concerned to follow a specially controlled diet to make up for the losses.

Bowel problems

These are also only seen in someone with extensive psoriasis. If the skin finds it is going short of the extra supplies it needs it may 'steal' them from tissues in other parts of the body such as the small bowel. If, as a result, the cells lining the small bowel become short of the nutrients they need their growth is altered and they become less able to absorb food. This can result in a kind of diarrhoea in which the faeces contain an abnormally high amount of fat. But I must emphasize that this is rarely a major problem and only happens in a very few cases.

Psychological effects

Having any kind of widespread skin condition can make you feel rotten, mentally as well as physically. When psoriasis affects large areas of the body you feel unattractive, and for young people in particular this can seriously affect relationships. In fact, most psoriatics seem to cope with this issue very well, form friendships in the usual way, and have normal lives. Not unnaturally, though, people with psoriasis often get periods of anxiety and depression. Sympathy from friends and family, reassurance from the doctor and proper treatment are all very important to help lighten the gloom. Meeting and talking over common problems with other psoriasis sufferers can also be a valuable way of easing depression and it could be worth your while to find out if there is a psoriasis group or society in your area (see chapter ten).

It is interesting that, in my experience at least, people with psoriasis seem to cope better with the psychological problems of their condition than do people with other skin diseases such as eczema. Psoriasis patients seem for the most part to be amazingly resilient people who cheerfully take life as it comes. This may perhaps be partly due to the fact that psoriasis is not generally an itchy disease and does not often affect the face. Both these things make it easier to adju   an some other skin problems. Another possibility, and one I   an to although there is no evidence for it, is that a psoriasis   s ability to accept his condition is an intrinsic part of his pe   y – just as the psoriasis is an inherent part of his physical ma   Whatever the reason, few psoriasis sufferers become seriou   ologically disturbed to the point of needing psychiatric tr   even though they may need occasional support and   nce from their doctors and their friends.

Another noticeable p   hat most of the psychological problems that people   iasis do experience improve dramatically as soon as   ve treatment is found. Their depressed state of mind would seem therefore to be simply a readily understandable reaction to the problems brought by the disease, not a basic feature of the condition or a factor in its cause. Just what does cause psoriasis is a question still swathed in mystery, but some of the answers that have so far been suggested are examined in the next chapter.

5

What Causes Psoriasis?

The cause of psoriasis is still not fully understood but it continues to be intensively researched. There are several factors which seem to influence it and I shall discuss them in this chapter, together with some of the things that have been mistakenly supposed to be connected with psoriasis. It is by gathering more and more information about the nature of the condition that we are most likely to come to explain its cause and perhaps from there discover the best way to cure or to prevent it.

Is it inherited?

It is well known that psoriasis tends to run in families. If one of your parents has the problem, you will have a one in four or five chance of developing it (much greater than the average likelihood). If both parents suffer from psoriasis the risk will increase to one in two. If one of a pair of twins gets it the other twin is particularly likely to get it as well. With identical twins there is a 70 per cent chance that, if one has psoriasis, the other one will too.

The fact that psoriasis can often not show itself until late in life does not rule out the possibility that it is an inherited condition. Many disorders that are inherited lie dormant for a number of years before showing themselves.

Other features of psoriasis, however, are not so easy to fit into the ordinary rules of heredity. To start with it is odd that, although in 90 per cent of cases where identical twins have the disease both of them will have it, there are still some cases where one twin develops it and the other does not. As both have identical genes it is hard to explain why, if psoriasis is an inherited condition, they should not always both follow exactly the same pattern.

Another puzzle is the way that, in about a third of all cases, psoriasis can occur out of the blue and afflict someone who has no family history of the disease at all. One theory is that this is due to what is called a new mutation. This means either that the genes that have been inherited only produce psoriasis under certain circumstances, or that there has been a freak alteration in the genes of one particular person. But there is no real evidence to support this idea in connection with psoriasis.

There are also oddities about the way in which psoriasis seems to be handed down from parent to child. It does not follow the same pattern as for many other traits we inherit such as eye colour. It seems to be more akin to the way we inherit general features such as height and intelligence, which result from a combination of several genetic factors in each parent.

Studies of the way psoriasis is inherited have been extensively researched, especially along the lines of investigating one particular factor in the disease known as HLA groupings (see page 31). From this type of research it has emerged that there are two 'types' of ordinary plaque-type psoriasis: one which tends to develop in young adults, and another that starts in the fifties or sixties. At the moment, while it is clear that the incidence of psoriasis is greater in some families than in others, we still do not fully understand whether or how it is directly inherited.

Two other possible explanations of the slightly unusual way psoriasis occurs within families are worth mentioning. The first is that psoriasis might not be one disorder but a collection of similar diseases, each of which has its own different pattern of inheritance. There is some evidence that this applies to nappy psoriasis and pustular psoriasis on the palms and soles. As pointed out above, there certainly seem to be two sorts of plaque-type psoriasis. If so, this would explain many of the current mysteries about why psoriasis seems to have some of the typical characteristics of an inherited disease but not others.

The second suggestion is that psoriasis might be some kind of viral infection. This would increase the risk of members of the same family getting it as they might transfer it to each other. This is not, of course, the same as inheriting the disease, and is a separate question which I shall now move on to discuss more fully.

Is it infectious?

In the ordinary sense, the answer to this is no. You don't get psoriasis by touching the spots or the scales – if you did, then all dermatologists would have it!

But, even though it is not an infection in the sense that, for example, tuberculosis is – in other words it is not something you can easily catch – there is a possibility that psoriasis might be due to some odd type of virus infection which will only attack certain people who just happen, for some reason, to be particularly susceptible to it. It is not a question of transferring the virus simply by contact – after all doctors and nurses frequently come into contact with psoriasis patients and they don't seem to be more likely to get the disease than anyone else.

Is it due to nerves or emotional factors?

A lot of people imagine that all rashes are in some way caused by how you are thinking of feeling – or, in popular speech, by your 'nerves'. 'Is it my nerves, doctor?' is a question I must hear half a dozen times a week in my dermatology clinic.

Until fairly recently many doctors believed that the intimate link between skin and a person's state of mind was the cause of skin disease. But that era has now passed and we tend today to demand a lot more evidence before we are ready to believe this.

Psoriasis is almost certainly not directly due to any psychological factors. But, having said this, it is true that any skin condition can be made worse by worry and depression and that psychological disturbance can even bring a skin problem out if you are already prone to it.

One clear example of this is the way that stress or worry can often affect psoriasis. It frequently seems to break out badly just before an examination, or after someone has suffered a sudden severe shock or bereavement. A typical example of the relation between stress and psoriasis would be the case of a patient called Geraldine who found her skin getting steadily worse as she became increasingly worried about her marriage. She suspected her husband was being unfaithful and he was starting to drink heavily which put her under additional mental strain. When eventually the couple got divorced, the improvement in her skin was rapid and noticeable.

Stressful circumstances can trigger off or highlight a whole range of physical diseases – not just skin complaints such as psoriasis, but heart disease, infections and even cancer. One suggestion is that the nerves in the skin actually release chemicals that start off the inflammation that leads to psoriasis. While there is no evidence that psoriasis can actually be caused by emotional disturbance, it can certainly be affected by the way you are feeling.

Is it due to your diet?

There is a popular belief that skin disorders are either due to or aggravated by eating the wrong things, and some of my patients ask me if they can improve their psoriasis by changing their diet. It has to be clearly stated that there is no established link between what people eat and the state of their psoriasis. It is a problem that can affect people on every kind of diet from the simplest to the most exotic.

A few years ago there used to be a special diet low in an amino acid known as trytophan which was sometimes recommended to psoriasis patients. But many scientific tests were done and they failed to prove that the diet helped with psoriasis in any way. As low trytophan diets are hard to devise in any case (for example, very few meats are low in trytophan other than turkey), it would be difficult as well as probably pointless to try to follow one.

One possible course that can sometimes improve psoriasis is to lose weight. Some of my patients who, for one reason or another, lost weight very rapidly, also found that their psoriasis cleared up. This may simply have been coincidence, but if you are anyway overweight it could be worth a try, as excess weight is unhealthy from any point of view. If you have flexural psoriasis it makes particular sense to try to stay fairly close to the normal weight for your height as any unnecessary folds of skin will be extra places for the psoriasis to strike.

What outside factors can make psoriasis worse?

Many things can make psoriasis flare up. I have mentioned the way a sudden shock or emotional upset can affect it, and there are also some kinds of infection that seem to make it worse. For example, if you get tonsillitis this can temporarily worsen your psoriasis, or can even appear to be what triggers it off. (This is particularly true of guttate psoriasis, as discussed in chapter two.)

If you suffer a cut or injury to your skin this can also have a bad effect, and sometimes make a patch of psoriasis spring up in a place where it hadn't previously appeared. Manual workers and other people whose hands come in for rough treatment sometimes find they get outbreaks of psoriasis on their hands as a result. Irritating your skin by scratching it can also bring out psoriasis, or make the patches sore, so this is something you should try to avoid doing.

Some people notice that their skin clears in the summer and then the patches break out again in the winter. Other people do not notice any changes from one season to another, and some even get worse when their skin is exposed to the sun.

One other question I am sometimes asked is whether having pets around the house can make the condition worse. The answer to this is no. Animals have no effect on the disease – and they cannot get psoriasis either.

Having looked at the general factors that can influence psoriasis in one way or another, many readers may be interested to know something about what is thought to cause the disease at a more fundamental level. The rest of this chapter, therefore, will describe, as briefly and simply as possible, some of the ideas that have been put forward by scientific researchers to explain the way psoriasis behaves and the reasons why certain people develop it.

The possible causes of psoriasis

There has been an enormous amount of work trying to find the cause of psoriasis. It really is a tough nut to crack, and we are still a long way off the answer. These are a few of the ideas being studied at the moment.

Is there a growth problem in skin cells?

The epidermal cells grow faster in psoriasis (page 17) and it has been suggested that this is because of an important inherited abnormality in the way that their growth is controlled. It has also been suggested that the way the epidermal cells mature is disturbed and that this abnormality is inherited. There is evidence that both growth and maturation are abnormal in psoriasis but we don't know whether these are the underlying problems or whether they are secondary to some other abnormality.

Is there a fundamental problem with the skin blood vessels?

The very small vessels (capillaries) near the skin surface look quite odd in psoriasis. They are wider and are much more curbed than normal. They are also leakier than normal. One theory suggests that these abnormal capillaries are the basis of the problem and start off the whole process.

The body's defence system

Most people will have come across the terms 'immune' and 'immunity' and will probably know that they refer to the body's system of defending itself. In the last ten years or so more and more attention has been paid to the way in which this system is involved in psoriasis.

An essential part of the body's immune system is that the tissues responsible for defence should be able to recognize what substances are part of the body (self) and what are not (non-self). When the system comes into contact with something that it does not recognize as self, it can then reject it. Sometimes however, for reasons we do not understand, the immune system makes a mistake and starts rejecting some of the body's own constituents. This sort of disorder is called auto-immune.

Recent evidence suggests that something like this may be happening in psoriasis. This whole area is extremely complex, and the scientists working on it have to use sophisticated techniques which are well beyond the scope of this book. But results so far have been encouraging, and I believe that exploration along these lines may well yield some important new insights into the disease in the future.

The white blood cells

Closely linked with the line of investigation I have just described, recent research is also being done in the way the white cells in the blood behave in psoriasis. It has been known for many years that these cells invade the affected patches of skin in a particular way. It now appears that there are some special substances found in the scales of psoriasis that attract white cells. (This is presumably why you sometimes get pus spots in connection with the condition.) Not only that, but there is also evidence to suggest that people with psoriasis have some particular factor in their blood that encourages these white cells to be much more active than usual. Both these discoveries open up new fields of investigation which might point to the underlying cause of psoriasis.

Links with other diseases

Psoriasis, as I mentioned on page 22, is known to be related in some ways to various types of arthritis. It shares with these diseases certain basic factors of body make-up which could provide us with clues to understanding it.

In the past twenty years research has shown that all of us have certain chemical characteristics which are found on the surfaces of all the cells in our bodies, and which can vary from one person to another. These chemical substances are known as HLA groupings (which stands for human leukocyte antigens). People who have the same HLA groupings share a number of genetic traits. They are more likely to accept organs and tissues from each other (for example, in kidney transplants) and they also tend to develop the same kinds of diseases as one another.

It has been found that there are a number of specific HLA patterns that people with psoriasis are more likely to have than a random group of the population. Moreover, some aspects of these patterns are shared by a substantial proportion of people who suffer from rheumatoid arthritis.

This kind of approach has been quite successful in working out relationships between diseases in other areas of medicine so it is not unreasonable to hope that it might come up with some significant results for psoriasis too.

In summary, it now seems that although psoriasis only develops in the skin it may not simply be a problem that arises in the skin itself. The underlying cause may turn out to be much more general and to involve basic chemical processess in our bodies. Intensive studies are being carried out, which make it more than likely that most of the details could be filled in within the next ten to fifteen years.

The future of research

I have not bothered to count the number of times so far I have had to write 'it is not known why . . .' or 'the reason for this is unknown'. So much about psoriasis is mysterious that I could easily fill a whole chapter simply by listing some of the things we *don't* know about it.

No kind of skin complaint is being more thoroughly researched than psoriasis, given the resources available. Besides the studies into the disease itself, we also depend enormously on advances in other fields (such as biochemistry and immunology) and on the development of new techniques for carrying out investigations. This means that professional research workers whose main interest is psoriasis must keep right up to date with science on a broad front as well as staying on top of their own subject.

Despite all the research work being done, progress is slow. This must, I think, lead us to ask whether the available resources are adequate or not. In my opinion the answer must be no. We are discussing a very common disease and one that causes untold unhappiness, ill health and economic loss. The number of investigators and the amounts of money available are far too small for the size of the problem. I sincerely hope that some of my readers will take this message to heart and do what they can to assist the research effort – not only by making donations. Publicity for the problem and agitation of the sometimes sluggish authorities can also play an important role.

The best prospect of finding new treatments rests with the basic research into the nature of psoriasis. Unless we strike lucky and hit on a cure by sheer chance we are totally dependent on the painstaking and costly efforts of the research scientist. Much good work has already been done and my guess is that we are nearer to finding a cure than we think we are.

In the meanwhile there are a number of treatments which, if they will not permanently cure, will at least relieve psoriasis in the short term and this is what I shall go on to discuss in the next four chapters.

6

Treatment – the Background

All the treatments we have for psoriasis at the moment are aimed simply at helping to clear the patches of affected skin rather than at eradicating the disease completely. Unfortunately almost no progress has so far been made in evolving a treatment of the second, more fundamental kind. This is sad but quite understandable. It is extremely difficult to design a basic, overall treatment until we know the real cause of the disease. It is rather like trying to swat a fly in a dark room with both your hands tied behind your back.

Having said this, there are a wide variety of treatments available to help with psoriasis, and I have tried in the next few chapters to describe them as comprehensively as possible. It is an important subject and one that should be interesting and relevant to most readers.

From the earlier chapters in this book you will already know that there are several types of psoriasis, and, not surprisingly, the treatment for each type differs. Treatment will also differ according to the stage of the disease, your age, whether you are being treated in hospital or as an outpatient and, to some extent, on your own and your doctor's individual preferences. I shall try to outline some general principles and to describe the various specific treatments that exist, both new and old. But first there are a few general points about treating psoriasis as a whole that are worth making.

You and your doctor

When you have finished reading the next few chapters you may feel you know everything there is to know about treating psoriasis. But this of course is not true. It is rather like, for example, thinking that once you know the general principles of how a jet engine works, you will be able to fly a plane. Apart from being stupid, this would actually be dangerous. And the same line of reasoning applies to medicine.

It takes a lot of skill and experience for a doctor to choose the treatment best suited to each patient. He has to balance the advantages and disadvantages of any given treatment with a special understanding of the particular problems of the person concerned. He also has to take into account the effects of the disease on other parts of the body and make due allowance for your skin type, age and weight. This is a delicate feat of judgement and one that even a skilled person would find hard to perform properly for himself. People who are directly and personally involved in a problem tend, naturally enough, to be the least able to take a clear and dispassionate view of it. And it is this detached approach that is needed in assessing the best way to deal with a disease such as psoriasis. In other words, there is no harm in learning all you can about the treatments available, but you must consult your doctor and allow him or her to make the decision on which one is best for you.

Testing new treatments

Many people wonder how a doctor discovers what particular treatments are likely to help psoriasis, and how different treatments become established. The answer is through what are known as clinical trials.

When a doctor gives you a drug in an attempt to relieve or cure a disease it is not like turning the key in a car ignition. There is no guarantee that the result will be just what was hoped for. In this sense all treatments are experiments – a fact that is particularly true of psoriasis because it is such a notoriously fickle condition. Several treatments may have to be tried before arriving at the right one.

New treatments for psoriasis are continually being devised, and they have to be tested in some way in order to find out how well they work. This is why your doctor may at some stage ask if you are willing to take part in a clinical trial – in other words a planned study aimed at discovering the effectiveness of a particular treatment.

There are various different types of clinical trial. One is known as an open study, which simply means that the doctor uses the treatment on a group of patients and keeps a record of the results. Another type is a blind controlled study, and in this case two groups are tested. The first group is given the new treatment and the second (the control group) is not, so that the results can then be compared. In a double blind controlled trial the second group is given a dummy or placebo treatment so that the patients and the doctor are both 'blind' and don't know who takes which drug. This guards against the possibility that the success or failure of the test might just be due to psychological factors rather than to the treatment itself.

Some people dislike the thought of being involved in a clinical trial. They may not want to be guinea pigs, or they may think the whole process is unfair. These are understandable reactions, but if all patients felt this way it would be much more difficult to find out how well any new treatment worked. Every effort is made to prevent people taking part in a clinical trial from suffering any inconvenience or danger, and the people who do agree to participate have the satisfaction of knowing that they may be helping to prove the value of a treatment that will afterwards bring relief to countless fellow sufferers, as well as to themselves. It is also important to know that all trials are now carefully considered by a special committee in each hospital. This is the research ethics committee, which takes great care to look after the patient's interests.

Models for research

Research into treatments for psoriasis would, of course, be much easier if there were some way we could test them out in a laboratory. If there were any animals who suffered from it, or if we could produce some material in a test tube that would respond in the same way as psoriasis does in man, the experiments would be much easier. In fact, although there are some animal 'models' they are not very good. Psoriasis does not happen spontaneously in any creature other than man. It is difficult to imitate psoriasis on the skin of rats or mice or other animals, and attempts to do this have so far not been very successful. There are also many people who believe all such animal experiments are immoral and wrong, and it is likely that the number of animals used in research will continue to decrease. It is also possible to do some studies in normal human volunteers without psoriasis – providing that they really are volunteers and that the research ethics committee I described above agrees.

Many people argue that the best model of all is a patch of psoriatic skin on a willing, human patient. They suggest that it is not only more ethical, but also more convenient and more appropriate from a scientific point of view, to use the human disease rather than to 'manufacture' it in animals or normal subjects – assuming of course that the experiments do not involve any danger for the human subjects. As tests for psoriasis are confined to only a small patch of skin, the hazard to the patient is very tiny indeed, and so there is a lot to be said in favour of this argument.

A point to remember

One of the first principles doctors are taught is summed up in the Latin motto *primum non nocere*, which translates freely as 'first and foremost, do no harm'. Psoriasis is not a serious health problem for most people, and it often improves of its own accord without any treatment at all. It would be quite unjustifiable to use any treatment that resulted in a worse problem than the disease itself.

7

Treatment with Ointments, Cream and Lotions

If you go to your doctor for the first time with a mild case of psoriasis, you are most likely to be offered an ointment, a cream or a lotion. As I have already said, it is especially easy for drugs in the form of creams or lotions to penetrate skin affected by psoriasis, and this means that treatment of this kind (sometimes known as a 'topical' treatment) often works very well.

How to use an ointment

The layer of cream or ointment you are putting on that actually does the most good is the part that is directly in contact with your skin, so it is wasteful as well as needlessly messy to pile it on in a thick coating. There is no point either in putting the preparation on areas of your skin that are free from psoriasis. Apply it accurately to the affected areas only, and rub it in gently so as to ensure that it makes thorough contact all over the patch of skin concerned.

Always follow the instructions that come with the ointment very carefully. This is especially important if the treatment also involves bathing and ultraviolet light therapy (see chapter nine). If the light rays have to get through a thick film of ointment before they reach your skin, you are unlikely to reap the full benefits of the treatment.

Remember that anything that comes into contact with the psoriasis patch can be absorbed very easily into your body. For this reason, if for no other, do not rub your psoriasis with anything and everything that well-meaning friends and relatives may offer you. If you are keen to try some ointment recommended by a friend, check back with your doctor first to make sure it will be alright.

If any of the treatments you are prescribed starts to irritate your skin instead of helping it, don't grimly persevere to the bitter end. Go back and let your doctor know that you are having trouble – he should be able to switch you over to something else that does not cause the same irritation. Incidentally, it is worth keeping a record of the names of the ointments, lotions and so forth that you have tried, and how they suited you. Remind the doctor if there are any of them you have had trouble with, so that he will know not to prescribe them on another occasion.

Do's and don'ts

- Always follow the instructions.
- Apply the preparation accurately to the patch of psoriasis.
- Rub it in gently to make good contact with the skin.
- Don't use lashings of the ointment when a thin film is all that is needed.
- Don't try other people's pet remedies until you have checked them with your doctor.
- Keep a record of your past treatments, and let your doctor know about any problems they gave you.

Preparations you can buy without a doctor's prescription

Many patients find that even a bland ointment with no special ingredients, such as Vaseline, can help to clear up or improve patches of psoriasis. Oily soaps, hand creams and bath oils sometimes help too.

It is hard to see why this should be so. One theory is that the Vaseline helps your skin to retain moisture better, and so softens the brittle, crumbling scales on the surface of an area of psoriasis. By stopping the skin from getting so dry it could also make it less likely to develop cracks. Other possibilities are that bland applications such as Vaseline may in some way help to slow down the rate at which the epidermal cells grow, or reduce the inflammation. Oily soaps or bath oils may help by leaving a protective, greasy film over the surface of your skin.

Whatever the reason, some of these bland creams and lotions do seem to have a good effect and it is simple common sense to make use of them. Even if you find that your psoriasis does not improve as a result of using Vaseline, at least you know that it is completely safe and has no harmful side-effects.

Treatments containing tar

Tar is a thick, black, oily liquid with a strong and distinctive smell. It is produced by distilling coal or wood. It had been used to treat psoriasis and various other skin conditions such as eczema for many years, and has often proved successful.

Why tar should help the skin to heal is a mystery. The pharmaceutical industry has spent huge amounts of money trying to discover just what it is in tar that makes it so effective, but so far without success. Tar contains many thousands of chemical substances and more than one of these may help the skin. It could also be that they have to work in a certain combination in order to have the healing effect, which would obviously complicate matters. No two batches of tar have exactly the same ingredients and some batches work better than others, so isolating the crucial constituents is, as you can imagine, a difficult task.

Crude coal tar can irritate the skin quite badly so it is rarely used in this form today. Instead you are likely to be given an ointment, cream, gel, shampoo or bath additive that contains a small amount of tar (anything from 0.5 to 5 per cent by weight). These should not irritate your skin, but some of them are messy, smelly and unpleasant to use. The modern ones tend to be much better in this respect than the old-fashioned kinds. Unfortunately tars have been accused of causing tumours and growths in mice. This has caused some concern but no evidence has been found that they cause such problems in humans.

Sometimes these preparations contain other ingredients as well as tar. For example, they may include some salicylic acid which seems to help banish the crumbly scale on top of a patch of psoriasis. Less commonly, hydrocortisone or other corticosteroids (see page 44) may be mixed in, but there is no proof yet that these creams are any more effective than ones which just contain tar.

How to use them

In the great majority of cases your psoriasis will be mild enough to be treated at home, and you will probably be given a cream or ointment to apply yourself. You will normally be advised to put it on once or twice a day, but this will depend on what it is and you should follow whatever instructions your doctor gives you. Continue with the treatment until the psoriasis has cleared and then stop. It is not a good idea to keep old jars of tar ointment (or for that matter any ointment or cream) with a view to using them again if the psoriasis comes back. The preparations can deteriorate with time so they may not work as well later on. More important, what you think is a recurrence of psoriasis may in fact be something else which will need a different treatment. It is always better to check back with your doctor to make sure.

There is one kind of treatment (called the Goeckermann regime after the American doctor who invented it) which uses tar ointments and baths in combination with ultraviolet light (see chapter nine). The tar seems to make people's skins more sensitive to light and so adds to the effectiveness of the ultraviolet therapy. This treatment is more easily carried out in hospital than at home. The sessions have to be repeated daily (or at least five times a week) over a period of two to three weeks, and the tar preparations used tend to be messy. However there are some day treatment centres for psoriasis where you can be given the Goeckermann treatment as an outpatient. At some you can go in the morning for a tar bath, ultraviolet lamp treatment and an application of the ointment and then go off to work as usual.

Avoiding mess Tar ointments tend to get on to your clothes and bed linen unless you do something to prevent this happening. The dark marks should wash out, but they can be rather annoying which is why parts of your body that are treated with these preparations are often protected with bandages. A simple tube-shaped bandage that stays in place and does not have to be wound on and off is often the most convenient. It is a lot easier to wash a few bandages than whole sets of clothes. If the areas being treated are on your abdomen or back, a set of cheap cotton underwear will carry out the same job as a bandage and keep your clothes free of mess. If you are being treated in hospital, the nurse may sprinkle a little dusting powder on to the treated area to cut down the mess, but this is not really necessary.

Treating your scalp The skin on your scalp is just as sensitive as that on your face, and ordinary tar preparations are a bit harsh for it. Special ointments and lotion have been developed for the scalp and are often quite effective. Lotions and creams containing corticosteroids are the most popular scalp treatments and are easy and not unpleasant to use. Older ointments tend to be made up of a mixture of traditional ingredients such as wood tar, sulphur, salicylic acid and coconut oil. They sometimes smell a bit odd and are not always popular with my patients!

Scalp preparation should be used sparingly, not plastered all over your scalp. Just dab a little of the preparation onto one of your fingertips and rub it gently into the psoriasis patch. There is no point in using it on areas not affected by psoriasis.

Another treatment sometimes recommended for psoriasis on the scalp is a tar shampoo. Some dermatologists are doubtful about whether these do any good, since shampoo only stays on your head for a short time. But if you have psoriasis on your scalp you will have to shampoo it frequently anyway – at least three times a week – to get rid of the treatments and scales, so you might as well use a tar shampoo (as long as you like the smell). More advice on looking after your hair is given in chapter ten.

How long do tar treatments take to work?

Used on its own, a tar preparation may take anything from three to six weeks to work. The Goeckermann regime works faster and can sometimes clear a patch of psoriasis within three weeks. The actual healing process is gradual, so don't expect the patches to vanish overnight. What you will see, if the treatment is working, is a gradual all-round improvement in the appearance of your skin. Bit by bit the redness, scaliness and roughness will all improve, until the spots slowly fade away altogether. Your skin may go on looking slightly red for a few weeks afterwards, but this too will disappear with time.

Dithranol

This is the name given to a highly reactive chemical compound that has some very powerful properties. It is also known as anthralin. Dithranol does have some disadvantages, as we shall see in a moment, but it is probably still the most effective treatment available for psoriasis. It is a synthetic derivative of the crude drug chrysarobin which occurs naturally in some plant extracts.

Exactly how dithranol works on psoriasis is not known, although a lot of research is going on to try to find the answer. One suggestion is that it somehow manages to damp down the excessive rate of growth in the cells of the epidermis, but this is not a complete explanation. Dithranol also seems to have a beneficial effect on the scales of psoriasis, and it may be that it counteracts the abnormal cell development that makes these scales. We still do not know whether it is the dithranol itself which is effective or some derivative formed in the skin. It is chemically a very unstable substance and so needs to be mixed with stabilizers to stop it deteriorating, particularly when in solution.

Dithranol is normally used as a cream or ointment. The amount of dithranol these preparations contain is usually something between 0.1 and 1 per cent by weight, but it can vary greatly and some ointments have as little as 0.01 per cent or as much as 10 per cent. People react to dithranol differently – some find it very irritating, only being able to tolerate very low concentrations.

The newest dithranol creams appear and feel quite pleasant to use. The greatest drawback to all dithranol preparations is that they leave stains on your clothing and bedclothes that cannot be washed off. So far no one has managed to come up with a dithranol product that entirely avoids this problem. Every pharmaceutical company dreams of producing a dithranol-like treatment that is cosmetically acceptable and that does not stain or burn. The creams produced in recent years are certainly a great improvement, but further advances are eagerly awaited.

Skin reactions to dithranol

The main difficulty with these ointments and creams is that dithranol can irritate or burn your skin. Whether it does so or not, and how badly, is something that varies from one person to another. Some people more or less turn bright red just as the sight of a jar of dithranol cream. Others can stand even the strongest concentrations without blinking. Unfortunately there is no way to tell in advance how anyone is going to react. People with blue eyes and light coloured hair (blonde or red) seem more vulnerable than those with fairly dark skin, but there are many exceptions to this rule. All the doctor can do is to adopt a cautious approach, using a system of trial and error. He will probably begin by prescribing a mild cream and then, if you do not show any bad reaction to this, may go on to try a stronger preparation.

It is obviously annoying and uncomfortable to get a severe reaction to dithranol, but it is not actually dangerous. I know a young woman who was accidentally given an ointment containing ten times as much dithranol as it should have done. She turned bright red as a result of using it, and felt quite sore. Even so, she recovered within two or three days simply by using Vaseline to soothe the irritated skin, and she suffered no long-term harm.

How to use dithranol

Not long ago dithranol was mainly used in hospital, and was combined with ultraviolet light treatment. This method is called the Ingram method after the doctor who pioneered it, and is still widely used. The stay in hospital may be anything between two and three weeks, and while you are there you get a treatment every day.

There are now also some excellent creams available which you can use at home. The newer creams tend to be less irritating than the older ones, but they do still have to be used with care. Follow whatever instructions the doctor gives you on how and when to apply the cream, and stop using it when the psoriasis has cleared up. Incidentally, dithranol can discolour your your hair if you use it on your scalp.

Once you have finished the treatment throw away any old jars or tubes you have left over. They do not keep well, and if you get any return of skin trouble you should go back to see your doctor again rather than dosing yourself with old medicines. With dithranol it is especially important never to use a cream or ointment passed on to you by someone else. It could turn out to be very much stronger than the one you are used to and could cause a severe inflammation.

Avoiding mess The brownish-purple stains that dithranol leaves on clothes, sheets and so forth cannot be washed out. If you are being treated in hospital, this may be their problem rather than yours, but if you are using a dithranol cream at home it is worth doing all you can to minimize the mess.

One way round the problem is to use what is termed 'short-contact treatment'. This is just what the name implies – the dithranol only stays on for an hour or so. In practice this means that the dithranol preparation is applied in the morning just after getting out of bed and kept on for one hour before being washed off. The short period of contact with the skin seems to be sufficient to have a therapeutic effect and the patient can remain active and out of a hospital bed.

It is wise to keep a pair of old sheets to use only when treating your psoriasis with dithranol, and to use a PVC protector underneath the bottom sheet to shield the mattress. A PVC pillowcase will help keep the pillow free of stains too.

It is difficult to prevent dithranol staining clothes. All you can do is to wear your least cherished items when using these preparations. A self-retaining bandage or a set of cotton underwear may help a bit, but the stain may seep through onto the clothes above. The treatment usually works within a matter of weeks, and then you can stop using the dithranol and put the marked clothes on one side again.

How long does dithranol take to work?

The Ingram method should work within two or three weeks, and dithranol used at home takes much the same time, or a bit longer.

One thing you may notice if you are using dithranol for the first time is that the skin around the patch of psoriasis being treated may turn a brownish-purple colour. This is nothing to worry about and does not mean the cream is irritating your skin. On the contrary, it seems to be an indication that the area is healing. Most of the discolouration disappears within ten days of stopping the treatment.

Corticosteroid creams and ointments

There is a group of hormones produced by our bodies called steroids (or corticosteroids), which have the effect of reducing inflammation. Corticosteroids can also be manmade substances. These resemble these natural steroids and have something of the same anti-inflammatory action. They first appeared in cream and ointment form during the 1950s and it soon became apparent that some of the more powerful among them could be effective in suppressing patches of psoriasis. They worked particularly well when they were put on under some kind of impervious plastic film. The corticosteroid creams available today not only work fast and effectively on patches of psoriasis, but also have the advantage that they are pleasant to use and quite acceptable cosmetically.

The problems of corticosteroids

The first drawback is a fundamental one. Although they suppress inflammation, corticosteroids do not seem to have any real healing effect on the skin. When you stop using the cream, the patches pop right back again. Worse still, they may come back more troublesome than they were before. Some dermatologists think that using the more potent corticosteroids may increase the risk that you will develop pustular psoriasis, which is one of the more unpleasant forms of the disease.

There are other serious potential hazards. In the first place, the corticosteroids applied to your skin do not just stay on the surface but get absorbed into your bloodstream. Since they so closely resemble the steroids we produce naturally, these synthetic corticosteroids may fool the body into cutting back its own output of steroids, including one vital hormone (called hydrocortisone) which we need in order to cope with stress. This cutback may not matter much as long as you are getting the corticosteroids to make up the loss, but when the treatment stops your body's reserves of hydrocortisone will be very low. This could be very dangerous, particularly if the body had to face up to some sudden emergency such as getting an infection or being involved in a road accident.

The risk of this happening is higher with corticosteroids taken by mouth than it is with the creams and ointments, but even so it poses a real threat.

If a large quantity of corticosteroids enters someone's body over a long period of time, there is also a remote risk that various other unpleasant side-effects will result. The patient may find that his physical appearance changes – his face may become rounder and redder, his arms and legs slim down and his stomach seem to swell. He is also in danger of getting high blood pressure and a type of diabetes, and may start to find that he bruises very easily.

All the risks I have described are slight and should not arise if the corticosteroids are properly used. Nonetheless they are real and worrying dangers, and your doctor is bound to consider them when deciding whether or not to prescribe you with corticosteroids.

Side-effects on the skin

As one might expect, corticosteroid creams have definite side-effects on the skin itself. The areas treated may produce a fine, downy growth of hair after some weeks or months, and may develop acne spots, particularly when the cream is used under an airtight adhesive bandage. The skin that has been treated tends to be prone to infection, and the patients also become more vulnerable to other common skin diseases such as ringworm and impetigo.

Where the corticosteroids have been applied the skin becomes abnormally thin. It may turn bright red or develop obvious stretch marks. Because it is so thin it is easily damaged. Even a minor injury can produce a nasty gash, and any knocks and bumps can lead to heavy bruising which takes a long time to fade.

These changes to the skin are more or less unavoidable if you use corticosteroid creams. Anyone who stays on this type of treatment over a period of weeks or months is bound to get these side-effects to some extent. Fortunately they do not usually cause any very serious problems, and the skin does eventually go back to normal when the treatment stops, apart from the stretch marks which tend to remain after all the other side-effects have disappeared. They are rather like the stretch marks people get during pregnancy or adolescence, except that they are slightly more noticeable.

In most cases the side-effects of corticosteroid treatment are more a nuisance to the patient than any real danger. They are not in my opinion the most worrying feature of this type of treatment. What does concern me far more is the way corticosteroids have come into such widespread use nowadays. They are powerful drugs and should be used cautiously, as I shall go on to discuss.

Vitamin D preparations Vitamin D and compounds like it (or 'analogues') have been found in recent years to be effective in psoriasis. One compound, known as calcipotriol, is already available in a cream (known as Dovonex in the UK) and has proved quite popular. Another is tacalcitol (known as Curatoderm in the UK). Others are being developed and will be available shortly. It is claimed that calcipotriol is as effective as dithranol. One advantage of these agents is that they don't stain, although they are quite irritating. Vitamin D's natural job in the body is to make sure that there is enough calcium around, and one potential problem with all vitamin D-type treatments is that they can raise the blood level of calcium to abnormally high levels. I did say it was a *potential* problem, because in practice calcipotriol has actually proved very safe to use.

Topical retinoids Retinoids are Vitamin A-like compounds (see page 55). Tazarotene is a new treatment (zorac). It is a gel which need only be used once a day and is quite effective in a short period of time, but it can irritate the skin.

How to use corticosteroids

As I have explained, corticosteroid creams work by suppressing all kinds of inflammation. What many people do not realize is that this may not always be a good thing. Inflammation is one of the ways our bodies fight infection. It is often a perfectly normal part of the process by which our tissues heal. By suppressing the inflammation we may find that we are allowing the infection to spread, and interfering with the normal healing process.

The way *not* to use corticosteroids is to turn to them automatically every time you get any kind of inflammation. It is not only people who store away old tubes of cream from previous treatments to dose themselves and their friends and family later on that are a danger here. It is also some over-eager doctors who take to prescribing them much too readily. Many people have been fooled into thinking that corticosteroids are the ideal answer to all skin disease, but this they certainly are not. Indeed, their popularity has probably done a lot to slow down the development of other new treatments for skin conditions.

Having said all this, I will admit that, even though corticosteroids are not my favourite treatment for psoriasis, I am not quite single-minded enough in my opposition to them to avoid prescribing them altogether. There are a few groups of patients for whom I think the benefits of corticosteroids may outweigh the drawbacks.

- People who have flexural psoriasis (affecting the sweaty parts of their bodies) and who have not found that any simpler treatments were effective.
- People with definitely diagnosed psoriasis of the scalp who have not been able to cure it with traditional remedies.
- People with unsightly patches on their faces or some areas on their genitalia, which have been firmly identified as psoriasis. In this case the kind of short-term improvement provided by corticosteroids is all that is wanted.

I also sometimes use corticosteroids combined with tazarotene, cal-cipotriol or tacalcitol preparations for cases of psoriasis that are not responding to other treatment. All I have to go on is my own observations of patients I have treated, but I think that combining the two treatments works better than using either of them on its own. This method also seems to cut down on the unpleasant side-effects of corticosteroids.

8

Pills, Potions and Injections

The idea of clearing up psoriasis simply by taking a pill has an obvious appeal. No messy ointments to stain clothes and sheets, no hours spent applying the stuff, no collection of jars and bottles to carry around or clutter up the bathroom – a safe, effective pill that had no unwanted side-effects would be a dream come true. Unfortunately we are still quite a way from turning the dream into a reality.

At the moment treatment with drugs is mainly used only for people with widespread psoriasis for whom ointments and creams in large quantities obviously become impractical. Sometimes pills are given in combination with creams, and sometimes the doctor will try to conquer the psoriasis with pills alone.

A medicine that you take by mouth or have injected affects all your body's systems and is often referred to as a systemic treatment for that reason. Special care has to be taken to see that this systemic treatment does no harm to any of the other organs it reaches besides the skin. You need to be especially careful too when taking systemic treatment, as misusing pills and potions is potentially a much more serious affair than being a bit careless in applying ointment. Before discussing the particular medicines available I shall therefore outline a few general points about using these kinds of treatment in the safest way.

Some do's and don'ts

- Follow your doctor's instructions exactly on how often to take the pills and how many to take. If he prescribes a complete course of treatment, make sure you finish the course.
- Keep all pills and medicines in a safe place out of the reach of children.
- Never keep pills in an unmarked container or one with the wrong label on it. You may think you will always remember what they are, but it is actually all too easy to forget.
- Let the doctor know if you get any problems such as sickness, diarrhoea, skin trouble and so on, that you think might be caused by the pills.
- If you are pregnant, remind your doctor about this before he

makes out your prescription and check that the medicine you are taking is safe to use in pregnancy.

- Check with your doctor whether there is anything you shouldn't do – such as operating machinery, driving or drinking alcohol – while you are taking the treatment.
- If you are taking corticosteroid pills, *never* stop without consulting your doctor.
- Never let anyone else 'try' your pills and never take any medicines prescribed for someone else.
- Don't keep a stock of half-finished medicines at the back of your store cupboard once you have stopped needing them. Take any left-over pills back to the pharmacist, and empty any remaining medicines in bottles down the toilet.

Some of the systemic treatments for psoriasis I shall discuss here are well established, others have fallen from favour, and a few are likely to become increasingly popular in the future. All of them are treatments you are only likely to be given if your psoriasis is quite bad and making you feel really ill. If you only suffer from the odd, mild patch this can usually be kept under control simply by using the creams and ointments described in the previous chapter.

Arsenic

This was part of the physician's stock in trade sixty years ago or more. Arsenic, dissolved in liquid and known as Fowler's solution, was prescribed in those days to treat 'anaemia', 'debility', 'fits' and skin diseases. In particular, it was supposed to have an almost miraculous healing effect on psoriasis.

It was given in very small quantities and so did not generally cause the type of violent poisoning so popular with writers of detective stories. But, after someone had been taking it for many years, it did cause serious problems – in particular a form of skin cancer and some other cancers too. The fact that these complications only developed after many years meant that they were not immediately linked with the arsenic treatment. There are no figures telling us how many people actually received arsenic treatment for long periods so we don't know exactly what proportion of them got unpleasant side-effects. And of course there is no way of telling for sure whether a particular person's cancer was due to his having taken arsenic previously, or to some other cause. But we do now have enough evidence to know that taking arsenic on a long-term basis is a definite danger to health.

Quite understandably, arsenic treatment has fallen out of favour. Nonetheless it is important to assess its value in context. All the systemic treatments available for psoriasis are 'poisonous' to some extent (although they do not do as much damage as arsenic over the long term). And, bearing this in mind, there is probably still a tiny case in favour of arsenic treatment under certain circumstances. If the patient concerned is over sixty-five and suffering from severe and disabling psoriasis which has not responded to other forms of treatment, arsenic, which only starts to have evil effects after many years, could be worth trying.

Corticosteroid medicines

As well as the corticosteroid creams and ointments I discussed in the last chapter, there are also corticosteroids that are taken by mouth or injected. These drugs, when taken systemically, suffer from all the same drawbacks as the corticosteroid creams and ointments, and are much more likely to produce the unpleasant side-effects I have already described (see page 45). In the doses generally given for psoriasis they may also cause problems such as stomach ulcers, acne, wasting of the muscles, and various psychological troubles.

In view of all these dangers, corticosteroid medicines are only used for psoriasis nowadays to treat very sick patients for whom no other treatment will work. Used in this sort of situation they can be 'miraculous' life-saving drugs, but in milder cases there is no justification for running all the risks involved in using them.

A special warning

If for any reason your doctor does prescribe systemic cortico-steroids, you must be sure to stick to the recommended dose *come what may*. If you stop taking the drug on your own account – say, because you feel sick – you could actually be endangering your life. As a result of the steroid treatment, your body may have cut back on its own production of certain important hormones such as hydro-cortisone, and it may not be able to cope with the stress of any sudden illness without it. In these circumstances it may be that you actually need more of the drug rather than less of it.

Methotrexate

This is a powerful drug, and is usually only given to people with severe psoriasis, for whom other treatments have proved too mild. It is undoubtedly an effective treatment for people with generalized psoriasis, or generalized pustular psoriasis (see chapter two). It also seems to help the unpleasant type of arthritis I described on page 22 and which sometimes afflicts patients with these severe forms of psoriasis.

Methotrexate is probably best known for its use in the treatment of various kinds of cancer, including leukaemia and Hodgkin's disease. (It is also sometimes used to stop the immune responses, for example when trying to reduce the risk that the body will reject a new kidney after a transplant operation). The reason why it works well for these kinds of conditions is because it stops the cells in our bodies from making a certain acid, and without this the cells do not divide and multiply so readily. In the case of psoriasis the drug seems to work by stopping the epidermal cells from growing as rapidly as they normally do in a patch of psoriatic skin.

Methotrexate was first used for psoriasis in the United States in the mid-1950s and it has since become an established treatment for people with serious forms of the disease. It used to be given as a pill which you took every day, but nowadays you are much more likely to be given it once a week, either in tablet form or as an injection, as it has proved safer this way.

How long does the treatment last?

Occasionally a short course of methotrexate lasting, say, less than six months, may be all that is needed to get you back to a more normal condition – at which point you can revert to the traditional creams and ointments to take care of the remaining patches. On the other hand, it may be necessary in some cases to go on taking the drug for a year or more before the tendency to generalized psoriasis has disappeared.

What are the side-effects?

Unfortunately, and as you might expect, this powerful drug does have some problems attached to it. If you are being treated with methotrexate you will have to have regular tests to make sure it is not causing any bad effects on your health.

One possible, but not too serious side-effect, is that you may get trouble with your stomach or bowels, as the drug can sometimes irritate these areas. If you find you are getting persistent feelings of sickness, indigestion or diarrhoea while taking the treatment, you should let your doctor know. Methotrexate can also affect the blood cells in the bone marrow, and you will be given frequent blood tests to check that this is not happening.

Effects on your liver

Unfortunately, there is no doubt that methotrexate can damage the liver. Whether it does or not depends on how much you take, how long you go on taking it, whether you take it regularly or only intermittently, and what state your liver is in to start with. A low dose, taken weekly for a fairly short period (for example, six months) by someone whose liver is healthy does not seem to cause problems.

You will, as I have said, be given regular blood tests while taking methotrexate, but this may not be enough to keep a close check on your liver. Many hospitals now like patients to have a liver biopsy before starting methotrexate treatment, and at intervals of a year to six months while they continue taking it. This means that the doctors can make quite sure what state your liver is in. This biopsy really is nothing to worry about and sounds much worse than it is. All that happens is that your side is numbed with an injection of local anaesthetic, and then a special kind of needle is used to take a tiny sample from your liver. Carried out in hospital this should not be either dangerous or even particularly uncomfortable, and it is the safest way to make sure that your liver does not suffer as a result of taking methotrexate.

It is well known that alcohol is bad for the liver, although that doesn't stop most of us from taking the occasional glass. As methotrexate can cause liver damage it is only sensible to try to cut out alcohol as far as possible while you are taking it. Strictly speaking you ought to avoid alcohol altogether until you stop taking the drug, but if this seems too much of a hardship for you, it will probably not do you any great harm to have the occasional glass of wine or beer – but no more!

Methotrexate and pregnancy

Methotrexate can have an effect on unborn children, and can even cause them to develop abnormalities. For this reason it is important that the drug should *never* be given to a woman who is or might be pregnant. It also means of course that any woman receiving methotrexate should take particular care to use really reliable methods of contraception throughout the time she is taking the drug, in order to avoid any possibility of becoming pregnant.

Can you get methotrexate ointments?

Some of you are probably wondering why, if methotrexate has such obvious side-effects when taken systemically, it isn't available in cream or ointment form. This is a thought that must have come to all of us interested in the treatment of psoriasis. In fact there have been many attempts to apply methotrexate successfully as a cream or ointment to the patches of psoriasis themselves. Unfortunately until recently all have failed, and why methotrexate should work when it is taken by mouth or injected but only with great difficulty when used directly on the skin itself is a real puzzle, and one that is occupying some of the best brains in psoriasis research at the time of writing.

Meanwhile, although it is not an ideal treatment for psoriasis, methotrexate has nonetheless given relief to many people, as well as stimulating the search for other even more effective drugs that might be less toxic. Recently progress has been made and a new, locally active methotrexate cream may soon be available.

Other drugs that damp down cell growth

Some of the other drugs that are frequently used to treat cancer have sometimes been tried on psoriasis. None is quite as effective as methotrexate and all have fairly similar side-effects. The side-effects are not always exactly the same, however, and so these other drugs sometimes come into their own for people who particularly want to avoid the effects of methotrexate. I know of one woman in her fifties, for example, who has really bad psoriasis and who has tried most of the available treatments over the years. Because her skin condition was making her really ill, she was given methotrexate, but as she enjoyed more than the occasional glass of alcohol and needed to continue the drug treatment over a long period, she began to develop liver damage. Fortunately it was possible to transfer her to another similar drug called razoxin which did less harm to her liver.

There are too many of these drugs to discuss here, but one – called nitrogen mustard – is worth a special mention. A lot of work has been done to try to make these anti-cell dividing drugs into creams and ointments, but nitrogen mustard has been the only one to date that has been successful. Unlike the others it seems to retain its beneficial effect even when painted on the skin as a liquid. I know of one major centre in the United States where this treatment is quite often given to patients with severe generalized psoriasis.

Possibilities for the future
Most current research work on the treatment of psoriasis involves the immunology of the disease. New treatments are being devel-

oped which change the immune response of the body and seem to help psoriasis.

Vitamin A and similar drugs

Vitamin A, or retinol, is a very interesting substance. It is found in dairy products such as milk, butter and cheese and in animal tissue (especially liver). It can also be manufactured by our bodies from something called carotene, which is found in plants – particularly red vegetables – such as carrots and tomatoes.

Vitamin A is necessary for many aspects of health. It helps our growth, the reproductive process, our vision and all our body surfaces, including our skin. Having too little vitamin A can cause several health problems, but this is only usually a risk in countries where undernourishment is still commonplace. Any reasonably nutritious diet will supply all the vitamin A our bodies need.

Perhaps because vitamin A was known to be important to keep the skin in good condition, it became quite routine about fifty years ago to prescribe it for people with acne, and a few other skin conditions – even if they were not actually suffering from a vitamin A deficiency. By all accounts some of the skin complaints did improve, but there were occasionally some unpleasant side-effects.

At the same time as doctors were using vitamin A in this way, scientists were making some interesting discoveries about how it worked on the skin. These discoveries led eventually to the appearance of new drugs, very closely related to vitamin A (the retinoids) but with greater potency compared to the side-effects of vitamin A. The first of these was vitamin A acid (all-trans-retinoic acid – also known as tretinoin), which is used in the form of a gel, cream or lotion to treat acne. It can also be helpful for psoriasis if it is used in conjunction with other treatments.

Other retinoid creams are being developed and tried for psoriasis and one of these, which is known by the fearsome reference AGN 190168, will probably be available in a year or two.

Retinoid drugs are mostly given by mouth for psoriasis. Two are known to be good for the disease – etretinate (trade name Tigason) and acitretin (trade name NeoTigason). The first of these is being replaced by the second, very similar, drug because of its advantages. How they work is mysterious but they certainly do have a good effect on patients with severe psoriasis.

Side-effects of retinoids

The retinoids are reserved for those with quite severe disease because of the side-effects of these drugs. It is worthwhile spending a few minutes on the side-effects as everyone who takes the retinoids should know about them. Most patients have minor inconveniences, such as drying of the lips, a temporary increased rate of hair loss and minor skin itchiness. These are minor problems and stop when the course of tablets is finished. Some patients have effects only visible from their blood, such as increased fats or chemical changes, suggesting that the liver is mildly inflamed. This is why blood tests should be done every six weeks or so. After taking the drugs for some years, odd changes in some of the bones have been found in a few patients.

Pregnancy The most serious problem with the retinoids is what happens if you are pregnant when you take the drug. Unfortunately, about half of babies born to mothers taking the drug have serious foetal abnormalities. This is why doctors are so insistent that women are having proper contraception (usually the pill) when on retinoids. In fact, in some countries women who can have children are not given retinoids for that reason.

Tigason, and to a lesser extent NeoTigason, is stored in body fat and takes a very long time to be eliminated after the drug has been stopped. For this reason contraception *must* be continued for two years after stopping – just to be on the safe side. This is only a problem for women, as there are no effects on men's sperm.

Because of all the potential problems and the experience required to give the right dose, the oral retinoid drugs can only be dispersed from a hospital pharmacy in the UK. Having said all this, most patients who are given oral retinoids do very well when taking them, and are not troubled by any of the side-effects. Certainly there are many patients who are very grateful for these vitamin-A-like drugs.

Sometimes retinoids are combined with other treatments, particularly ultraviolet light treatments such as PUVA (see page 62).

Cyclosporin

This potent drug has only recently been introduced for the treatment of psoriasis although it has been used for patients receiving organ transplants for some years. It suppresses the body's immunological reactions and this is why it is used in patients receiving new kidneys or hearts – it stops these organs being rejected. Whether it is this 'immunosuppressive' activity that is responsible for its effects in psoriasis is not settled, but it seems quite likely. As with the other oral treatments, it is reserved for patients with severe psoriasis because of the side-effects. With cyclosporin the side-effects are on the kidneys and on the blood pressure. The kidneys can become quite irritated and the blood pressure can go up significantly. This is why blood pressure is taken and blood and urine tests are performed each time you come to the clinic.

New cyclosporin-type drugs which suppress the immune system are being developed and almost certainly will be available soon.

9

Sun Treatments and Ultraviolet Light

Patients with psoriasis have known for many years that exposure to the sun can be very helpful in clearing their rash. It does not apply to every case, but it is certainly true for the majority. It does not follow that there is no psoriasis in sunny places like Australia, southern Africa or the sun belt of the United States. Rather curiously, there is as much psoriasis in sunny climates as in colder ones, although psoriasis sufferers may be able to get rid of their skin trouble more quickly in sunny areas.

A whole group of treatments for psoriasis has grown up around the beneficial effect of sunlight on psoriasis. To understand some of these treatments properly, we first need to learn a bit more about the sun's rays.

The sun's light

The sun radiates energy in the form of waves. These light waves we can see can be split up by a prism into a spectrum of red, orange, yellow, green, blue, indigo and violet colours. Radiant light energy of a shorter wavelength than violet is known as ultraviolet light. This is the part of the sun's energy that has important effects upon our skin.

Ultraviolet light can itself be split up into three groups, A, B and C, according to its wavelength. It is the middle group of waves, ultraviolet light B (or UVB), that makes up the most important part of the sun's ultraviolet light as far as our skin is concerned. It is UVB that causes most sunburn, and UVB too that helps heal psoriasis (possibly by damping down the high growth rate of the cells within the epidermis). Some UVA reaches us in sunlight, but it has much less effect on our skin than UVB. Very little UVC gets through the ozone and the atmosphere surrounding the earth to reach us at all.

If you happen to be one of the many people whose psoriasis is helped by exposure to the sun, it does not follow that you should bare your skin to the sun at every chance you get. There are good reasons for being cautious, and not regarding sunlight as an unmixed blessing, as we shall see.

Sun and your skin

Our skin protects itself from the burning rays of the sun by turning brown. The brown colouring (called melanin) is produced within the epidermis and absorbs the ultraviolet light, which helps prevent it from burning the skin. People with fair skin produce less melanin than swarthy, dark-skinned people, and this is why they burn more easily when exposed to the sun. Black-skinned people produce a lot of melanin, but even the darkest skin will burn eventually if it is exposed to too much ultraviolet light. This is the first reason for caution in sunbathing. Quite apart from being painful, severe sunburn can actually make your psoriasis worse rather than better.

The harm the sun can do to your skin does not stop at burning. Sunlight also damages the lower, tough part of the skin known as the collagen, so that after several years of exposure the skin starts to lose its suppleness and elasticity. The result is that the pursuit of a gorgeous tan in your youth can leave you looking like a wrinkled prune by middle age.

An even worse risk to the really dedicated sun worshipper is that of developing all types of skin cancer. This is a common disease in really sunny parts of the world where it has become a major public health problem. But it is certainly not restricted to these countries, as there is a serious increasing risk of skin cancer of all types in most parts of the world, including Europe. This is mainly because of increased leisure time and the cheapness of holiday travel. The decrease in the ozone layer may also have something to do with the problem.

In any event, the bottom line is, the more you are exposed to the sun's rays, the greater the risk of developing one of the skin cancers.

It should be clear by now that it simply does not make sense to try to treat your psoriasis by toasting your skin unmercifully. Not only your appearance but your health may suffer in the long run if you overdo things. If you want to try sun treatment (and if you are lucky enough to live in a place where the climate makes sunbathing feasible) you should take a careful, planned approach to it. Here are some general guidelines to follow:

Guide to sunbathing

- Check up with your doctor before you start to make sure that any medicines you are taking will not make you extra-sensitive to sunlight.
- Wipe off any ointments or creams you have been using to treat your psoriasis.

- Start cautiously. On the first day you should spend no more than ten minutes in the sun.
- Increase the length of exposure gradually, adding ten minutes a day until you reach a maximum of one hour.
- Stop once your psoriasis has improved.
- Always remember that too much exposure to sunlight will damage rather than help your skin.

Using suncreams

Some substances absorb (or reflect) ultraviolet light or prevent its rays from passing through them. If you wear an ointment or cream containing these substances, you can give your skin some protection against sunburn. This is the basis of most suncreams and lotions.

How much protection any cream gives depends on what it contains (as well, of course, as on how carefully and how often you apply it). The 'sun protection factor' that many creams quote gives an indication of how thoroughly they will shield your skin. The higher the factor, the greater the protection. Fair-skinned people should look for a cream with a protection factor or six or more, since they are likely to burn easily. But remember that even a high-protection preparation will not stop you burning if the sun is very strong.

Most creams tend to wash off in water, so it is wise to reapply them after a swim. The creams also tend to rub off on towels, seats, rugs and so on, so it is best to reapply them every few hours even if you stay on dry land and are out of the sun for part of the time.

Spas and health resorts

In some parts of the world health resorts and spas have become such a recognized treatment for psoriasis that you can actually claim back some of the cost of visiting one from the state. Even in countries where this is not the case, there is widespread and growing appreciation of the numerous health benefits to be gained from a period in the relaxing atmosphere of a health spa.

The spas where most psoriasis patients go are either on the Dead Sea in Israel, or in Lanzarote in the Canary Islands. What these places can offer in abundance is sunlight. This, in fact, is the key to the whole value of a spa for psoriasis, which is why the treatment is sometimes called climatotherapy.

The resort in En Boqeq on the Dead Sea is the most popular of all the climatotherapy centres. As well as the outstanding beauty of its surroundings, this resort can offer sunlight with a quite special quality. Because En Boqeq is well below sea level, the sun's rays have to travel through a thicker belt of the earth's atmosphere before they reach the ground. As a result, most of the harmful UVB is filtered out. The rays of ultraviolet light that are left seem to be rather gentler and not as likely to burn the skin as ordinary sunlight.

The qualities of the water in the Dead Sea may also play a part in helping psoriasis. It is unusually salty and contains all kinds of minerals and other solids. In fact the water is so full of dissolved solids that it is almost impossible to sink in it. It is quite possible that this special water has unusual healing properties, although this has not been proved. At any rate, it is fun to bathe in and certainly does no harm.

Bathing and sunbathing at a special spa among others with similar complaints also sometimes has the advantage that people with psoriasis feel less self-conscious there than they do when sunbathing on public beaches.

Expert medical supervision is another aspect of treatment at a health spa. This, combined with the change of scene, rest, relaxation and agreeable surroundings, can all play some role in improving psoriasis. It would be interesting to know whether the good effects of health spas last longer than those produced by routine treatment, and whether more people benefit from health spas than from other treatments. Unfortunately we don't have answers to these questions at the moment.

It is a surprising fact that the cost of treatment at these spas often compares very favourably with that of a similar length of time spent in hospital. Some countries even make special arrangements to send people who need intensive treatment for psoriasis to the Dead Sea rather than to a local hospital because it actually works out cheaper!

Sunlamps and psoriasis

Some of us don't have much opportunity to expose our skin to natural sunlight, because we don't see strong sun very often. Some psoriasis patients in this situation try to give their skin artificial sun therapy by using a sunlamp. These devices, which produce ultraviolet light at the turn of a switch, can certainly help people who have psoriasis, but ideally you should not use them without medical supervision. In inexpert hands they can cause a lot of damage.

Why you need to take care

- Sunlamps produce mainly UVB, the type of ultraviolet light that causes sunburn. You can end up with very painful burns if you use the lamp in a foolhardy way.

- Sunlamps damage the skin in just the same way as sunlight. The ultraviolet light attacks the collagen within the dermis, and makes the skin look old before its time. And, like any other form of ultraviolet light, it increases the risk of skin cancer.
- Like all electrical devices, a sunlamp can give you an electric shock if it is treated carelessly or wrongly wired. In addition, the lamp can become so hot that it would burn anyone who touched it by accident, and it could start a fire if used too close to anything inflammable.
- Medicines can affect the way your skin reacts to ultraviolet light, and so can ointments and creams. Using a sunlamp without your doctor's advice while you are taking one of these sensitizing treatments is asking for trouble.

How to use a sunlamp

It should go without saying that if you decide to go ahead and use a sunlamp at home anyway, you *must* follow the instructions carefully on how to use your particular lamp. Incidentally, if you have psoriasis over much of your body, a small lamp will be very little good to you, since the ultraviolet light it produces will only reach a small area of your skin in any one session.

It is worth remembering two more points about sunlamps. First, the effect of the ultraviolet light on your skin increases more than proportionately as you get nearer the lamp. For example, if you halve the distance between you and the lamp, this will boost the amount of ultraviolet light hitting your skin not by double, but by four times. So you need to pay attention to the distance you are from the lamp as well as to the length of time you spend under it. In the second place, the older a sunlamp gets, the less powerful it becomes. (Some manufacturers supply information about this along with the instructions on how to use the lamp.) This means that you must take extra care if you ever use someone else's lamp. Even if it looks just like the one you normally use, it is not safe to assume the two lamps are equally powerful. The one you borrow might be newer than yours and you could end up getting burnt.

Sunlamps give the best results when they are used under the right conditions and with the right care. If they are used ignorantly or carelessly they do far more harm than good.

PUVA (photochemotherapy using ultra-violet A-type light)

Among the chemicals that make our skin more sensitive to light are some substances called psoralens, which are found in plants. Their medical potential is not a new discovery (they are even said to have been used in ancient Egypt), but their use in treating psoriasis started only twenty-five years ago.

How PUVA works

Psoralens make the skin particularly sensitive to the longer wavelengths of ultraviolet light (UVA). What happens in PUVA (pronounced poo-va), is that you are given a psoralen preparation and then, two hours later, exposed to UVA form a special lamp. The dose of the psoralen and the length of exposure to the light rays both have to be carefully regulated to produce PUVA's healing effect.

There is no real explanation for how PUVA helps psoriasis. Our best guess to date is that, by greatly magnifying the effects of ultraviolet rays, the psoralens damp down the high rate of growth of the cells within the epidermis that is such a feature of psoriasis. Several groups of researchers are trying to lift the mystery that surrounds how PUVA works. Attention is being paid not only to the impact it has on the skin, but also to how it might affect the body's immune system or the white cells. Ways of treating psoriasis with other kinds of ultraviolet light as well as UVA are also being explored. But my own guess is that these investigations, while possibly helpful in the short run, are unlikely to produce important advances in the treatment of psoriasis.

How you get PUVA

PUVA is not available everywhere. If it is available near you, and your doctor thinks it is the right treatment in your case, you may have to go into hospital for your first course of treatment to make sure that everything is closely monitored.

The dose of psoralens is usally taken as a tablet, but a few dermatologists prefer to treat only the skin rather than the whole body by putting a solution of psoralen into bath water or by painting the PUVA solution directly on to the psoriasis patches. 'Tablet'-type PUVA is more convenient but not necessarily more effective.

The PUVA lamps used are somewhat different from ordinary sun-lamps. They are often built into boxes, rather like shower cabinets, into which you step for treatment. Alternatively, sets of lamps may be arranged above a table for you to lie on. There are smaller PUVA units that can be used to treat just your hands or feet.

Some patients dislike the rather claustrophobic feeling of being shut up inside the PUVA cabinet, and some elderly people find it difficult and uncomfortable to stand up inside the cabinet for the time the treatment session takes. I have even known one or two extremely large patients who couldn't fit into the PUVA cabinet at all – but they were definitely exceptional!

The length of the treatment session really has to be established for each patient as people differ in how sensitive they are to ultraviolet light. You will probably start off with short sessions which will get gradually longer as it becomes clear how your skin is reacting. Sessions are not likely to last more than twenty minutes. It is important to wear dark-tinted goggles while the treatment is going on and for twenty-four hours after to prevent damage to your eyes from the sun's UVA. The goggles should be tested to make sure they block UVA.

How long does the treatment take?

Your first course of PUVA may take three or four weeks – a lot depends on how your skin reacts to it. Once the psoriasis has cleared, the PUVA treatment may be continued once or twice a week in the hope that this will stop the problem coming back, but the fact that there has been considerable disquiet concerning the safety of PUVA (as I shall go on to discuss), must make all concerned quite cautious about continuing the treatment on a long-term basis.

How effective is PUVA?

When it was first introduced a few years ago, PUVA was hailed as a new wonder treatment for psoriasis. Now, after some twenty years of painstaking assessment, it seems that PUVA's virtues were definitely overrated. It does help psoriasis, but neither faster nor more permanently than traditional remedies such as tar ointments and dithranol.

PUVA has undoubtedly proved very popular with patients, and it is easy to see why. It does not involve any messy, evil-smelling creams and ointments. There are no stains to ruin clothes and bed linen. The golden suntan PUVA users develop is attractive and fashionable too. It is scarcely surprising that, even if PUVA is no more effective than older remedies for psoriasis, patients should be keen to try it. But there is less enthusiasm for PUVA among the medical profession and there are sound reasons for this caution.

What are the drawbacks?

Some of the disadvantages of PUVA (although not the most crucial ones) are economic. It is a relatively expensive form of treatment, and its results hardly seem to justify the high cost of administering it. The skilled staff who are needed to supervize the use of the PUVA lamps might possibly be able to use their time better by giving a different kind of therapy to a larger number of people.

The more serious drawbacks to PUVA are the doubts about its safety. Neither in the United States nor in Britain has official approval been given to its use.

One risk that is being particularly seriously considered is that exposure to ultraviolet light may speed up the development of skin cancer. One survey in the United States showed that patients who had a lot of PUVA had about a ten times' risk of skin cancer after some ten years. Not all surveys have agreed with this greatly increased risk and the skin cancers are quite easy to treat. Even so, it would seem prudent to be aware of the possibility and to cut down on the amount of extra sun exposure. For this reason some PUVA centres will not treat fair-skinned patients at all, as these people tend to be at the greatest risk of developing skin growths.

It is also possible that some of the UVA will reach the blood close to the surface of your skin. This could lower the body's resistance to infections while the treatment is going on and for a short time after it is over. There may also be other long-term risks that we have not yet been able to identify.

A more immediate hazard is that your skin could get burnt. It is extremely difficult to calculate the precise dose of UVA that will be right for a particular person. Too high a dose can lead to severe burns, and these do happen from time to time even with the most expert supervision.

Finally, the risks of PUVA may not be confined to the patients themselves. Some medical workers are reluctant to operate the equipment on the grounds that the ultraviolet light to which they themselves get exposed presents a health hazard.

Narrow Band UVB

This is a new type of ultraviolet treatment which is claimed to work faster than PUVA. The name comes from the very narrow waveband of the lamps used (312nm). My experience is that it is quite effective – but it is early days to say how useful it will be.

10

Living With Psoriasis

Anyone reading this book must have realized by now that psoriasis covers a very wide variety of conditions. These range equally widely in their severity. At one end of the spectrum is the person who has the odd patch of psoriasis on his body which causes so little trouble that he scarcely notices it and needs no treatment at all. In the middle there is the patient whose psoriasis flares up in several places a couple of times a year but dies down again quickly when treated. Right at the far end of the spectrum are the few unlucky people whose lives may be really disrupted by their condition – people with generalized or severe and widespread psoriasis that needs long-term medical treatment.

So far as everyday life goes, people with very mild, intermittent psoriasis should have few or no problems at all. Happily, the majority of sufferers are in just this position, and my hope is that more and more will become so as new treatments for psoriasis are developed.

Unfortunately no dermatologist can rule out the possibility that, even if you have mild psoriasis, it might not suddenly flare up to present you with a whole range of problems – some trivial, some more bothering. If this should happen, I hope the material in this chapter could make coping with these problems easier.

I find it encouraging to see how well even people with fairly bad psoriasis can come to terms with the problems it can cause. One young woman I treated came to see me about three weeks before she was due to get married. She had quite a lot of psoriasis on her body and legs as well as some on her face (which is uncommon). I thought she might be worried about how her psoriasis would affect love-making and about it upsetting the sexual side of her marriage – but not a bit of it! She and her fiancé had very sensibly discussed this possibility and put the matter to the test, so she had good reason to feel confident on that score. Her only worry was that the psoriasis on her face would make her look in the wedding photographs as if she had had too much to drink! We managed to clear her face in time, and the marriage went ahead without any further doubts or problems. People who have a positive attitude like this towards life seem to cope splendidly even with the problems that only quite bad psoriasis can cause.

Of course, there are psoriasis sufferers whose experiences are less encouraging. They may have difficulties at school, trouble settling down and finding a job and worries about relationships with the opposite sex. They may find it difficult to persuade unsympathetic employers to give them the time off work that they need to get treatment for their psoriasis. Lack of self-confidence in dealing with other people may make them feel lonely and isolated. In an unusually severe case, the patient may experience all these problems. A more typical picture, however, would be of someone who runs into difficulties now and then as a result of his psoriasis, occasionally feels depressed about his condition, but most of the time manages to come to terms with it fairly well.

Many of you reading this book will have had personal experience of the problems associated with psoriasis, but I believe it is worthwhile going through them one by one and seeing what positive things can be done to help to overcome them.

Taking care of your appearance

One of the things that sometimes makes it hard to maintain high morale when you have psoriasis is knowing that your appearance is suffering as a result of it. Most people devise their own ways of improving matters, but other people's tips can be very valuable. Here are some of the things you can do to help yourself look good in spite of your rash. Exchanging ideas with other fellow sufferers is a good way to find out more.

Your hair

Psoriasis on the scalp is one of the commonest causes of concern. As well as being uncomfortable, it can produce showers of white flakes that look like a bad case of dandruff. It is bound to be annoying to cope with, but there are a few tips that may help.

- Go for a short hairstyle, if you can find one that suits you. You will have to wash your hair often to get rid of the scale and the old ointment, and long hair or styles that need fiddly setting may end up driving you mad.
- Shampooing too often can make your hair lose condition and your scalp feel sore. On the other hand, not shampooing enough will allow the scale on the patches of psoriasis to build up. It is important to find the right balance for you. I usually recommend that men should shampoo their hair every other day, in the morning. Women with long hair may find this is too much trouble

and have to make do with washing it less frequently. Some dermatologists recommend that you use a shampoo containing tar as this is sometimes thought to help the psoriasis.

- If you go to a hairdresser, find one who knows about psoriasis and is not reluctant to cut or style your hair when you have patches of it on your scalp. Your local psoriasis association (see page 75) may be able to suggest a good hairdresser in your area.
- Women who develop cracks in the skin of their scalp should avoid having a perm or colouring their hair until the trouble is improved. The harsh solutions used to perm and colour could irritate the scalp condition and make it worse. When the scalp is clear, it may still be worthwhile looking for as mild a perm or colouring as possible.
- Wear light coloured clothes as the scales will show less.

Your face

It is unusual to develop psoriasis patches on the face, so most people do not have to cope with this particular problem. A woman can disguise a rash on her face by using a good cover-up cream under her ordinary face make-up. This should not do your skin any harm and (especially on a special occasion) it can make you look and feel a lot better. Incidentally, it seems that many ordinary brands of make-up are no more likely to irritate sensitive skin than the so-called hypoallergenic brands – so there is probably no need to choose one of the latter, which tend to be pricey.

Your arms, legs and body

Psoriasis on these areas is usually not a major problem in terms of appearance, since it can usually be covered up with clothes. Women may find the same sort of cover-up cream discussed above useful to disguise patches on their legs, if these show through their stockings. The less sheer the stockings, of course, the better they will conceal the psoriasis.

In a fairly cool climate, you may be able to get away without stripping off even if you play sports. Tracksuits are often just as acceptable as shorts for outdoor games, and you can take advantage of this if you are really reluctant to show your arms and legs.

What should you use to wash with?

It does not greatly matter which sort of soap you use, but oily and emollient soaps and cleansers are best. All you need is to find one that does not irritate your skin and that helps get rid of the scale. Some dermatologists believe that it is helpful to use some sort of tar in the bath and, as long as this does not irritate your skin, it is quite a good idea. Your doctor should be able to give you the tar liquid to put in the bath to serve this purpose. Also, as I mentioned in chapter seven, ordinary bath oils can sometimes help psoriasis by leaving a protective film over the surface of your skin. Otherwise any fairly bland, simple soap or emulsifying ointment should be perfectly alright.

Your clothes

The particular problem here, of course, is the ointments and creams that many psoriasis sufferers have to use to treat their skin. If you have to use creams that stain, such as dithranol, then it obviously makes sense to keep a special set of underclothes to wear while the treatment is going on, so that the rest of your clothes will be protected. If the cream is merely messy and not staining, then wearing something light and easy to wash between the psoriasis patch and your ordinary clothes may cut down on the amount of washing to be done.

Some of the newer dithranol creams are claimed to be nicer to use than the older versions, but they don't avoid mess altogether. Until an effective, non-staining ointment is developed, most psoriasis sufferers can really only try to grin and bear the inconvenience of traditional remedies.

Choosing clothes that disguise patches of psoriasis is, as I mentioned earlier, not usually difficult. Most people do not find that their hands or face are affected. And if, for example, you get patches on your arms which means you don't want to wear sleeveless garments, it is still possible, even in hot weather, to find cool clothes with long sleeves that cover your arms. Only in a few instances, such as when you are wearing swimwear, is it likely to be difficult to disguise the patches. But even then you can wear a light shirt over your bikini or bathing trunks to hide areas of psoriasis on your arms or back.

Of course if you can overcome your self-consciousness about your condition you will feel free to wear any clothes you like. It is, after all, quite common to have a blemish of one kind or another on the skin and many people learn to come to terms with this and do not mind whether or not it shows. But this is of course easier said than done and it takes a good deal of courage to overcome shyness.

Getting enough rest

Psoriasis tends to flare up in any sort of stressful situation, regardless of whether the stress is physical, mental or emotional. So one of the most useful things you can do is try to cut down the stress you are normally exposed to. It is often difficult to know how to go about this, but one thing that certainly sometimes helps to relieve feelings of anger, guilt or anxiety is talking over your problems with someone else. Many family doctors are skilled at this sort of discussion, and it may also be possible to raise some of the issues that are bothering you with a group of fellow psoriasis sufferers.

The second essential is to get enough rest. Many diseases improve spontaneously if the patient manages to spend enough time resting, and psoriasis is no exception. One of the reasons why a spell in hospital can produce an improvement in psoriasis is probably simply that hospitalization forces you to rest more. If you are at home you could get some of the same benefits from laying aside time during the day to sit quietly and relax.

Can psoriasis affect pregnancy?

There is no reason why a woman with psoriasis should not have a perfectly normal pregnancy. And pregnancy does not normally affect the state of psoriasis either – except that some women find their skin improves. Uncommonly it may get a little worse late on in the pregnancy or after the child has been born.

As I mentioned in chapter eight, it is very important that a pregnant woman should never take the anti-psoriasis drugs methotrexate or the retinoids Tigason or NeoTigason as these can harm the child. Most other psoriasis medicines are quite safe to take during pregnancy, but you should always check up on this with your doctor.

Is alcohol bad for psoriasis?

My own impression is that people with psoriasis often seem to have happy, outgoing personalities. One feature of this otherwise excellent tendency is less of an asset – it sometimes brings with it a fondness for alcohol. Problems associated with drink seem in my experience to turn up more frequently among patients with psoriasis than among those with other long-term disorders (although I may turn out to be quite wrong about this). It may be that people with psoriasis 'drink to forget'. Or they may just be happy types who enjoy the social side of drinking. A more intriguing possibility is that psoriasis might somehow alter their body chemistry so that alcohol becomes especially appealing to them.

Alcohol does not have an adverse affect on the psoriasis as such, although too much can of course bring a number of other problems. One effect it can have is to produce a mild inflammation of the liver, and it is not uncommon to find that patients with severe psoriasis cannot be given methotrexate because their livers have been damaged in this way. As I mentioned on page 53, you should do your best to avoid alcohol if you are taking a course of methotrexate because this drug can also have an effect on your liver. The same is true, but to a lesser extent, with the retinoid drugs.

Is smoking bad for psoriasis?

The answer to this is most emphatically 'Yes'. Smoking is bad for you anyway, but it seems there is an enormously increased risk of developing pustular psoriasis if you are a smoker. We do not know why, but it may be that there is a good chemical reason why this is the case. Whether giving up smoking will improve psoriasis is not established, but it can only help.

Protecting your skin

Avoiding injury

Grazes or minor injuries tend to make psoriasis break out or get worse, so it is as well to take extra care to avoid damaging your skin. Most everyday tasks should not do any harm – it is only if you actually cut or graze yourself that psoriasis may get worse. Doing rough sports, or jobs that might hurt your hands can be a problem. Patches of psoriasis tend to bleed very easily even after a minor injury. Creams or protective clothing are the only real defence against this but, if these are not enough, you may feel you have to avoid doing the activities that irritate the psoriasis.

Around the house

It is a good idea to wear thick gardening gloves for work outside to protect your skin from injury by thorns or prickles and to prevent soiling. It is also a good idea to wear protective PVC gloves for washing up and other tasks that involve putting your hands in water. Water, soap suds, detergents and so forth will not actually make your psoriasis worse, but they tend to dry out the skin and make it more likely to crack. If you do wear PVC gloves for any length of time you should use a handcream underneath them, as the gloves tend to make your hands sweat which dries them out. Regular use of handcream is anyway a good way to help keep your skin supple and less liable to crack.

People with psoriasis on their hands who want to use their fingers for jobs such as typing, handling papers or operating manual controls may find that using lotions and creams makes their fingers too greasy. In this case it can sometimes help to wear a light pair of cotton gloves. The same principle can be applied to patches of psoriasis on other parts of your body. If you put on the cream or ointment first you can then cover it up with a bandage or light piece of clothing to prevent the greasiness from causing problems. It is as well to make sure this protective covering is something easily washable as it will quickly become stained and need to be frequently changed.

At night the creams and ointments may mark the bedclothes. You should be able to get protective plastic sheets and pillowcases to put under your regular ones so that the stain will not go through to the pillow or mattress. Housework, even at the best of times, is not much fun and all the extra washing you have to do when using ointments to treat your psoriasis can make it a real chore. Anything you can do to reduce this burden is obviously well worthwhile.

Going on holiday

I have already referred to the benefits people with psoriasis can get from a period of rest, and taking a break to go on holiday can have the same good effects. Whether you choose a relaxing or an energetic holiday, it can be very helpful just to get away from the stresses of your everyday life.

If your psoriasis is quite bad there may be some kinds of rough, adventurous holidays that it would be difficult for you to manage, but this is something that will obviously vary enormously from one person to another – depending on how widespread your psoriasis is and how much treatment it needs. Choosing a holiday that will suit you is entirely a matter for your individual judgement and preferences. If you do need reassuring that you will not be at risk of making your condition worse your own doctor will be the best able to give you individual advice.

As far as beach holidays go, these do of course have some positive advantages for people with psoriasis. Judicious sunbathing (see chapter nine) can improve your skin, and many people also find that swimming in salt water is beneficial. The only thing that is sometimes a problem is if you are self-conscious about revealing your psoriasis on a crowded beach. You may find that if you start off by sunbathing somewhere private – say, in the garden at home or on a private balcony – this might help you to get over some of the self-consciousness. Otherwise it will be a question of finding ways to cover up the affected patches of skin – or, if you are very lucky, discovering a piece of beach you can have all to yourself!

Relationships

It takes a lot of courage to go out and meet new people and make friends when you have a noticeable skin disease. The fear of being rebuffed can lead psoriasis sufferers to keep themselves to themselves to such an extent that they end up lonely and isolated.

One of the most helpful things you can do in this situation is to find some fellow sufferers with whom you can talk over your feelings. The knowledge that others are fighting just the same problems as you can be very reassuring and dispel feelings of isolation. Details about how to get in touch with other psoriasis patients are given on page 75.

It is possible that you will find it easier to forget about your psoriasis if you meet others in the context of some definite activity – a sport or hobby, for example – that keeps your mind on what you are doing. This may help you take a more relaxed attitude towards other people, and hence help them to accept you too.

What really would help most people with very prominent psoriasis is, of course, recognition on the part of other people that fear and revulsion are simply not appropriate responses to a non-infectious, non-contagious skin condition like psoriasis. This is almost entirely a question of educating the general public into a better awareness of what psoriasis is. This is something that all of us who have an interest in psoriasis – patients, doctors, family and friends – can do something about, by putting pressure on health educators and administrators to devote more of their resources to skin disease. The result in the long run might be to change the community's whole attitude towards skin disease patients, and very much improve their chances of living otherwise normal lives.

Does psoriasis lead to sexual problems?

Skin and hair are important parts of the body so far as attracting the opposite sex is concerned. If they are in some way abnormal, not only may there be an actual problem finding a partner but the person involved may magnify the problem out of all proportion and lose that essential part of sexual attractiveness – confidence.

Coping with this difficulty is largely a matter of recognizing its nature. After all, psoriasis very rarely affects the ability to make love. In the unusual cases where there are a few small patches of psoriasis on a man's penis or on the woman's vulva, treatment usually shifts the rash quite easily. Small patches elsewhere can be masked with cover-up cream, if the patient feels they matter a lot.

As a rule, having a few patches of psoriasis on the body does not seem to interfere with either party's enjoyment of sex. If large areas of skin are involved, however, there are potential difficulties. If so much psoriasis is present that either partner feels reluctant to make love, it is important that the couple should get sexual counselling to help them through this trouble. Simply discussing problems with the family doctor may help by reassuring you and producing a more relaxed attitude towards the problem. Tension is bound to make any sexual difficulties worse.

Doctors as a group are possibly rather slow to recognize the importance of problems like this for the patient's general health, and some are bashful about offering suggestions. Luckily attitudes are changing, and nowadays help should be available to any psoriasis sufferer in need of guidance on sexual matters.

Success at work

At the time I am writing this, unemployment is a particular problem. To keep a job it is especially important to have a good attendance record and to perform well. In today's difficult economic circumstances employers can hardly be expected to give work to those who for some reason or another do not seem able to work successfully.

Having said this, I must point out right away that in general there is no reason why psoriasis should prevent you from doing well in any trade or profession, despite the problems you may have from time to time. I know one man in his late forties who has persistent generalized psoriasis and painful arthritis into the bargain who works as a heavy goods vehicle driver. He works the normal hours of the job, loads, unloads and looks after his truck – all completely successfully. Another generalized psoriasis sufferer I know has a highly successful career in business which involves him in a lot of travel and many contacts with people all over the country. He is something of a whizz-kid and his business is growing from strength to strength in spite of the fact that he suffers from an unusually severe form of psoriasis. It seems that, given the right approach to work, psoriasis should not be any barrier to success.

Nonetheless people with psoriasis may have to overcome special obstacles in the path of their careers. Some jobs involve taking a medical examination before you start work, and where this happens the applicant with psoriasis may have a hard time convincing the employer that his skin condition is no reason for turning him down. The armed forces seem particularly unenlightened in this respect, and it is rare for someone with more than mild psoriasis to be able to make his or her career in the armed services.

People with a lot of psoriasis on their hands or feet can find certain sorts of work difficult. Psoriasis in these areas tends to produce cracks in the skin that can make using the hands or walking painful – so work that requires fine hand movements or frequent trips over rough ground is likely to cause the patient a lot of discomfort. The only thing to do in this situation, unfortunately, is to stop this type of work until the hands have healed. Anyone who has this problem from time to time may find it worthwhile to wear protective gloves wherever possible to protect the skin from injuries that could trigger off an attack of psoriasis. Generous applications of handcream may help too, by keeping the scaling skin as pliable and elastic as possible.

It ought to be inconceivable that someone who has a benign skin disease on a small area of his body should lose out at work because of it. Unfortunately ignorance and prejudice do still exist and the only way to dispel this is to educate the general public as well as possible about psoriasis so that they no longer view it as something to fear or distrust. This is one of the many valuable roles that can be carried out by psoriasis groups which can operate locally, nationally and internationally, to increase understanding of the disease for sufferers and non-sufferers alike.

Psoriasis associations and societies

These have sprung up all over the world. The organizations have slightly different names in different countries (The Psoriasis Association in the United Kingdom, the National Psoriasis Foundation in the United States) but they share essentially the same purpose and philosophy. A new society has recently been formed for those who have the arthritis associated with psoriasis. This is called The Psoriatic Arthropathy Support Group. The various national societies belong to an international organization, the International Federation of Psoriasis Associations. This enables the different groups to keep in touch with each other and keeps them up to date with what is going on in other parts of the world. The addresses of the head offices of these societies are given in the Useful Addresses section at the end of this book.

These societies generally aim to give support to people who have psoriasis and to promote knowledge and understanding of the disease. At grass-roots level they consist of local clubs, societies or chapters, often based in a local hospital or clinic.

How they can help you

I believe local groups of psoriasis patients are of immense importance, and I think they do far more than just act as a forum where people can exchange experiences and swop ideas, valuable though this is. In my opinion, joining in with the group's activities can do a lot to reduce the feeling of loneliness that so many psoriasis patients experience.

A wide range of activities goes on, often orientated towards fund raising: parties, dances, concerts, bring-and-buy sales, fetes, lectures, and various sponsored activities. People seem to enter into them with great enthusiasm. Even more important than their fund raising aspect, in my opinion, is the feeling of camaraderie they produce among the members.

The associations as pressure groups

Some people I know (including, regrettably, some doctors) seem to be afraid that when patients group together in societies and associations like this they become 'organized to demand' special treatments or facilities. If this were so, in my opinion it might not be such a bad thing in some cases. Where adequate facilities for psoriasis patients do not exist, then a bit of well-directed pressure from the psoriasis groups might achieve some improvements. In any case, I think that fears that these groups will try to agitate for the wrong things or in the wrong way are quite groundless. Most groups have good contacts with doctors, dermatologists, social agencies and so forth, and they talk out their problems with help from these sources. The good sense I have heard talked at such meetings makes an aggressive approach unlikely.

An example of the way psoriasis groups can use pressure effectively is their success in persuading some local swimming pools to allocate their members a special time to use the pool. This has been a real pleasure to many patients who were either too embarrassed by their psoriasis to bathe with the general public or were prevented from doing so by a rule forbidding those with skin diseases to use the pool when other people were there.

Educating the public

Many of the problems touched on in this chapter could be prevented if people in general knew more about psoriasis and what it involves. The national societies have an important role to play in this area, by pressing for more funds to be spent on educating the public about skin disease, and by disseminating information about psoriasis. The newsletters or magazines that some of these societies produce tend to have a wider readership than those who are themselves suffering from the disease, and can be excellent.

All in all, the psoriasis societies can give patients the kind of assistance and support that no doctor, social worker, relative or friend can supply quite as effectively. What they need above all if they are to work well is your support. Join a psoriasis society if you can and help it to help all psoriasis sufferers.

Other sources of help

Many psoriasis patients will be able to turn to the community for certain kinds of help with their problems. The exact sort of help available differs from country to country. If you are in doubt about whether or not you might qualify for this kind of assistance, your local psoriasis society may be able to help you with information and advice.

One problem that occurs quite often is that a patient whose job involves heavy manual work develops cracks on his hands that make it painful for him to do his job. If it is impossible to persuade the employer that the patient should be moved temporarily to a more suitable type of work, a community job guidance service may be able to put other kind of work the patient's way. Medical social workers can be tremendously good at solving this type of problem, and doctors should be ready to take advantage of the service they offer.

Occasionally accommodation causes the psoriasis sufferer trouble. One elderly woman I know had extensive psoriasis and arthritis that meant she needed special bathing and toilet facilities. A social worker helped her to get structural alterations made to her tiny, old-fashioned house to cater for these special needs.

This is the type of difficulty that psoriasis patients can often find help with, once they become aware of the range of sources of help that they may call on.

11

Questions and Answers

I hope that, if you have already read the rest of this book, it will have answered most of your questions about psoriasis. But I have found that there are several particular doubts and anxieties that crop up again and again among people who have just been told that they have the disease, and I thought it would be worthwhile going through them briefly here. Fuller details are given on all these topics in the earlier chapters, but anyone who wants quick answers to some of the basic questions most often asked about psoriasis may find it helpful to have them set out separately in this section.

What is psoriasis?

Psoriasis is a long-lasting or recurring skin disorder. We don't know its cause and at the moment there is no cure. It only affects patches of the skin and usually does not cause ill health. The psoriasis patches are actually thickenings of the outer layer of the skin. The cells in this part grow more rapidly than normal and cause the crumbly scale you see on top of a psoriasis patch.

Is psoriasis a common disease?

Yes, it is very common. About two per cent of the population have it. Some types of psoriasis are much more common than others. The most usual kind (plaque-type) accounts for about 95 per cent of all cases. Pustular psoriasis is much less common, and generalized psoriasis (all over the body) is quite rare – I would estimate that it only affects one or two per cent of the total number of people with psoriasis.

Is it infectious?

No. You can't 'catch' psoriasis or transfer it to someone else just by touching the scales. Infectious skin diseases used to be common many years ago and some people still fear that they can catch them by contact, but nowadays infectious skin diseases are a rarity.

Is it caused by stress?

No. We don't know the cause of psoriasis but it is almost certainly not due to any psychological disorder. It is of course true, on the other hand, that all skin problems can be made worse by worry and emotional disturbance, and that severe psoriasis can sometimes make you feel anxious or depressed.

Is it due to my diet?

No. Psoriasis occurs among people on all kinds of diet – reducing, fattening, high fat, low fat, vegetarian, vegan, organic, etc. What is more, no particular diet seems any better than another for treatment. In general terms it is better to avoid becoming over-weight – if only for aesthetic reasons!

Why did I get it?

I don't know the answer to this one. The best answer we have is that you may have been born with a tendency to develop psoriasis, inherited from your parents.

Will it spread?

It might do and it might not, but usually it doesn't. Very often psoriasis sticks to certain places (in particular the knees, elbows, back and scalp) and causes no more than a nuisance. It is very uncommon for it to affect large areas of the skin or cause general ill health.

How long will it last?

Unfortunately there is no way of knowing in any particular case whether the psoriasis will grumble on for a long time or whether it will go away of its own accord. Often it does clear up, but it is impossible to predict how long it will take to do so.

Will I go bald?

No. Psoriasis does not make you go bald even though one of its favourite areas is the scalp. If you do lose some hair this loss is certainly *not* permanent.

Is scratching bad for psoriasis?

Not particularly, but it can make it feel sore or bring out more patches in places you have scratched.

Will it affect my sex life?

No, psoriasis should not affect your sex life. If you or your partner are worried about sexual problems your family doctor should be able to help you. The most important thing is for both partners to understand something about the disease and overcome any fears they may have about it, then it should not interfere with a normal and happy sex life at all.

Will psoriasis affect my pregnancy?

No, it should not. There is no reason why a woman with psoriasis should not have a completely normal pregnancy. Sometimes the pregnancy has an effect on the skin disease and makes it get slightly better or, towards the end of the pregnancy, rather worse. But most often there is no change at all.

Will my child get psoriasis?

It is impossible to predict this. About one third of all people with psoriasis have one parent with the disease, and their probability of getting it doubles if both parents have psoriasis. It is uncommon for someone to develop the disease before their late teens or early twenties.

Why are all the tests necessary?

A good question! Mostly they are designed to tell your doctor whether what you have is really psoriasis. Sometimes your doctor will ask you to cooperate in a research test. It is up to you to decide whether to help or not, but remember that psoriasis won't be beaten without a lot more research.

Will the sun help my psoriasis?

Probably yes. But this is really quite a complex question. The part of sunlight that helps psoriasis is the ultraviolet light which can also be produced by special lamps and a treatment called PUVA (see page 62). Ultraviolet light treatment is often given together with creams or ointments. Unfortunately ultraviolet light can have bad effects as well as gone ones and so it must always be used cautiously and under supervision. If your skin gets burnt as a result of using it, this can actually make your psoriasis worse rather than better. It is interesting that psoriasis is just as common in places with sunny climates as in cloudy, north-west Europe.

How often should I shampoo?

As often as you feel you need to, which may be as much as every other day, in order to stop the build-up of scale on the psoriatic patches. Some dermatologists like tar to be included in the shampoo as this could help the condition.

What should I wash with?

Any bland soap or cleansing lotion is perfectly alright. Choose one that will help get rid of the scale and that does not irritate your skin. Tar liquids to put in your bath can sometimes have a beneficial effect.

How does dithranol ointment work?

Nobody is sure. It may be that its actions are different. It stops the rapid growth of epidermal cells or somehow changes the way the epidermal cells change into the horny layer.

How do Vitamin D analogues and retinoids work?

We are not certain, but we think that they help epidermal cells develop normally. They may also damp down the inflammation.

How do methotrexate, the retinoids or cyclosporin work?

Nobody knows for sure. They may all work in different ways. Methotrexate seems to cut down the rate at which the epidermal cells divide. The retinoids (Tigason and NeoTigason) may alter the way the cells mature and grow. Cyclosporin seems to damp down the body's immune response and this may alter the degree of inflammation in the affected skin.

Is any research being done on psoriasis?

Yes, quite a lot – but not enough. The shortage of funds and facilities for studies of skin diseases make life difficult for the professional researcher. The lack of public awareness about psoriasis also hinders progress.

What prospect is there for a cure in psoriasis?

This is a difficult question. Ask me again in ten years! My guess is that we are much nearer than we think we are. Recent progress in the understanding of psoriasis makes it more likely that we will have a more permanent way of treating the condition, but how long this will take is difficult to predict.

Should I join a psoriasis association or society?

Yes, most emphatically. These groups help enormously. Give them your support!

Useful Addresses

Any of the following organizations can tell you where to get help:

UNITED STATES

The American Dermatological Association
Medical College of Georgia
Augusta
Georgia 30902

The National Psoriasis Foundation
6443 SW Beaverton Highway
3210 Portland
Oregon 97221

The Psoriasis Association
107 Vista Del Grande
San Carlos
California 94070

BRITAIN

The Psoriasis Association
7 Milton Street
Northampton NN2 7JG
(Tel: 01604 711129)

The Psoriatic Arthropathy Support Group
136 High Street
Bushey, Watford
Hertfordshire WD2 3DJ
(Tel: 01923 672837)

CANADA

Psoriasis Education Research Centre
60 Grosvenor Street
Toronto
Ontario M5S 1B6

AUSTRALIA

The Skin and Psoriasis Foundation
PO Box 228
Collins Street
3000 Melbourne

NEW ZEALAND

The Auckland Psoriasis Society
PO Box 3062
Auckland 1

Index